Anti Inflammatory Diet

The Simple Plan - Proven To Fight Pain & Disease With Whole Foods & Natural Remedies

Table of Contents

Introduction

I want to thank and congratulate you for purchasing the book, "Anti Inflammatory Diet: The Simple Plan - Proven To Fight Pain & Disease With Whole Foods & Natural Remedies".

This book contains proven steps and strategies on how to fight inflammation, discomfort and disease through food and natural remedies.

This book will show you why you need to follow a special diet that helps minimise inflammatory conditions such as rheumatoid arthritis. This is also helpful if you're trying to manage autoimmune diseases such as lupus. The diet includes avoiding certain kinds of food particularly fatty food, oils, and refined sugars. Completely avoiding these foods in the first try might be a bit difficult so you need to ease into it.

Chapter 1 will introduce you to what is an Anti-inflammatory diet. There are also examples of possible ailments and kind of lifestyle you follow that may cause the inflammatory issues.

In chapter 2, you will have access to a list of food to eat and avoid. The list is by no means exhaustive because there are thousands of food items out there. You can just use this list to get started and then use online resources to build your own list. In the next chapter, you will be given some Anti-Inflammatory Diet tips. Here, you will finally have the answers to your questions if you should eat this kind of food or not. There are times when you can eat certain food even if the category they belong to is in the pro-inflammation list. It all depends on your body's capability to decipher it as a stressor or not.

There are natural remedies that assist in relieving you from pain brought about by inflammation. Know more of these remedies in chapter 5.

Chapter 5 is a bonus chapter that will show you a sampler for the anti-inflammatory diet — a 5-day meal plan.

Break your habits. Learn how to eliminate the bad substances that are causing inflammation in your body. If you cannot terminate the relationship immediately, take them in moderation. You will see a different you in a month's time that is healthier and stronger without the inflammation.

Good luck and thanks again for purchasing this book. I hope you enjoy it!

Chapter 1
Anti Inflammatory Diet – An Overview

Inflammation in itself is not always a bad thing. In fact, it is an important mechanism of the body's immune system. It enables the body to heal. It usually occurs during injury or attack by microorganisms; the local heat and swelling, as well and the accompanying symptoms only mean that your body is aware that something is wrong and it's doing its best to send more nourishment and antibodies to the affected area.

However, chronic inflammation such as in the case of rheumatoid arthritis and other autoimmune conditions is not at all a good thing. It is also related to the development of Alzheimer's, Parkinson's, certain heart conditions, and even certain forms of cancer.

There are certain kinds of food that make the condition worse, if not trigger it. Food items that have high sugar and saturated fat content can cause an overactive immune system, and in turn trigger inflammation, which is manifested in joint pain, fatigue, and blood vessel damage.

The average American diet in particular is extremely pro-inflammatory. It features high a lot of calories from fat, making your body prone to inflammation. This is especially the case with fried food and other dishes prepared with high amounts of fatty oils and seeds such as partially hydrogenated vegetable oils and margarine that have high Omega 6 content. This fatty acid helps create more hormones that trigger inflammation.

By reducing your intake of the high inflammatory food in your diet, you can reduce inflammation. Not only is it healthy; it also typically does not involve heavily processed food and it is rich in antioxidants. As an added bonus, it could help you lose weight.

Symptoms of Inflammation Syndrome

So how do you know its high time to start maintaining an anti-inflammatory diet regimen? It might help to watch out for symptoms. It can be difficult to detect the problems right away. The only way for you to feel something is not right is when the inflammation causes your organs to lose its function. This is where the anti-inflammatory diet comes in as a preventive antidote to future diseases.

Exercise Difficulties

Patients have a difficult time completing an hour of vigorous exercise. They often complain of sharp pain in their lower extremities or swollen joints. If you are having this problem, it is best to do moderate intensity exercises with 5-minute intervals.

Constant and Lingering Pain

Patients complain of a dull ache on both sides of their bodies as well as below the waist. The duration of the pain lasts for at least 3 months.

Irritable Bowel Syndrome

Some patients experience frequent abdominal pain, abdominal gas and constipation.

Note that patients who experience chronic inflammation need to undergo different tests before pinpointing what treatment will work for them. The treatment is dependent on a particular symptom to provide relief instead of a cure. This may involve getting enough rest to allow the body to truly heal, antidepressants to correct hormone imbalances, and the Anti-Inflammatory diet.

Causes

Do you have the following ailments or been diagnosed with such? These are the top causes of inflammatory issues.

Emphysema

Bronchitis

Stroke

Cancer

Fibromyalgia

Diabetes Type 2

Alzheimer's disease

Dementia

Rheumatoid Arthritis

Asthma

Cancer

Colon ulcers

Risk Factors (lifestyle)

Inflammation signals pain and discomfort. You may experience the causes mentioned above mainly because of the lifestyle or condition of life that you follow.

Obesity

Chronic pain (headaches, joint and muscle soreness, back pain)

Minimal or no exercise

Physical and mental lethargy

Regular or excessive intake of anti-inflammatory medicines

Regular intake of refined sugar and carbonated beverages

Regular consumption of grain-based products

Regular consumption of grain-fed meat

Regular intake of dairy products (unless dairy substitutes)

Chapter 2
What To Eat And What Not To Eat

What You Need To Avoid

These pro-inflammatory foods are present in a standard American diet. They are one of the reasons that inflammation is present in the body.

Safflower, peanut, corn, sunflower and soybean oils: These are inflammatory foods because they have high Omega-6 fats content that metabolise hormones that trigger inflammation

Fried food: Trans-fat is present in processed or fast foods, especially those that are fried. It is best to avoid eating this at all time.

Food high in refined carbohydrates, which are present in flour, sugar and foods high on the GI or Glycemic Index. Examples of such food include cake, pretzels, and chips. These food help elevate glucose levels and insulin.

Fatty food particularly those with high saturated fat content such as butter, cream, chicken skin, fatty meat and high fat cheeses.

Anti-Inflammatory Food To Eat

Know the right kind of food to reduce your chances of having inflammatory issues. They are all-natural and easy to find in the market.

Fish

Choose food that is low in cholesterol and sodium. These two components trigger inflammation. As discussed in the introduction, you need to eat food that is high in protein as well. The way to add protein in your diet is to switch to fish. They are high in omega-3 fatty acid. Start looking for halibut, cod, snapper, salmon, and bass recipes

Oil

Instead of using canola or vegetable oil, reach out for olive oil when you prepare fried fish. You should also try extra virgin variety for salads. Olive oil is rich in omega-9 fatty acid. According to research, omega-9 is rich in nutrients that help reduce inflammation.

Nuts And Fruits

It is advisable to eat fruits and nuts in between meals such as in almonds, hazelnuts, walnuts and sunflower seeds. They are high in omega-3 fatty acids. Fruits can always take the place of chips and cookies since they contain antioxidants. Eat these foods to fight the free radicals in the body that often cause cellular damage. The most common types of filling fruits are pineapples, strawberries, blueberries, cherries and apples.

Garlic

Garlic helps to ease inflammation. Although it does not smell good especially when eaten in public, garlic has anti-inflammatory components that can be eaten raw, in capsules or be eaten as part of a viand.

Herbs

Promote healing and good health by adding herbs to your food. They are a good source of antioxidants that help reduce pain and swelling. The next time you prepare your meals, make sure to include thyme, basil, oregano, and rosemary.

Chocolate

Here is good news for sweet lovers! Chocolate is one of the best foods to eat in an anti-inflammatory diet. You can use the 70 percent pure cocoa variety and not worry about insulin spikes.

Moderate your chocolate intake by choosing the dark and very dark chocolates instead of the sweet milk chocolates.

Carbohydrate sources

Instead of baked goods made with refined flour, you should opt for more winter squashes, beans, sweet potatoes, whole-grain bread, and brown rice.

Vegetables

The anti-inflammatory diet allows you to eat 5 smaller meals in a day, Eating raw vegetables actually gives you a balanced measurement of nutrients, fibre and water that will keep you from feeling hungry. These vegetables do not lose their flavours and force you to add too much sugar and salt just to get the taste you want. Indigestion happens when you over stimulate your intestines by the condiments you add.

Preparing salads take as much as 15 minutes or less versus traditional recipes that need half a day to complete. Did you know that super foods have more nutrients than most other foods? They contain minerals, nutrients and vitamins that prevent disease. Take note of these super foods so you can add them in your Anti-Inflammatory diet.

Maca

It is rich in protein, carbohydrates and fatty acids. And not to mention, Maca has high levels of phytonutrients, minerals and vitamins. It boosts energy levels, libido, and fertility in both men and women. What is great about this superfood is that it also boosts immunity and lowers high blood pressure.

Wheatgrass Juice

It has 30 excellent iron, magnesium, zinc, calcium and potassium content. Wheatgrass is a detoxifier that eliminates odour in the body as well as reduces cravings, which lead you to overeat.

Bee Pollen

This superfood has 96 nutrients and is a great source of energy. Bee pollen slows down aging and reduced one's cholesterol levels. Aside from that, this super food improves sperm count in men, boosts one's immune system and improves endurance. The best thing about the bee pollen is that it helps in weight loss by burning body fat.

Chapter 3
24 Anti-Inflammatory Diet Tips

Tip #1: Include Important Food In Your Daily Menu

There is no single meal plan for Anti-Inflammatory Diet. In fact, it is generally considered as a general wellness diet, which means it can be pretty flexible. However, it is advisable to keep the following as staples - oatmeal toasts with yogurt and berries for breakfast, fish recipes such as tuna salad with grain bread, and more fruits for lunch, and turkey pasta, salad and butter less apple pies or bread for dinner. Snack time will be worth looking forward to since it includes 1 oz. of dark chocolate and 4 whole walnuts.

Tip #2: Eliminate Sugar, Grains, Legumes, Dairy And Legumes For 1 Month.

The Anti-Inflammatory diet could be even more effective if you start with a detox diet for a month. Allow your body to accept its absence for 30 days and after that, you will feel the difference.

Refer to this 1-month detox as your mind and body-conditioning program in order to accept the Anti-Inflammatory diet.

Tip #3: Eliminate Unhealthy Fat In Your Diet

Bid farewell to food that is rich in Omega-6 Fatty acids. Make it a point to check the labels if you go shopping and search for this. However, if you are to dine outside, do not order food that requires margarine or deep-frying to prepare. Opt for restaurants that use olive oil in frying if you absolutely have to.

Tip #4: Thank The Heavens For Monounsaturated Oils

It is time to smile and thank the heavens for extra-virgin olive oil, olive oil and the wonderful Omega-3 Fatty acids. You can also use fish oil, flaxseed oil, walnut oil and hempseed oil. Whether you will toss it in a salad or sauté vegetables, these oils are now your new BFFs.

Tip #5: Say Goodbye To Unhealthy Carbohydrates

Try to avoid commercially produced muffins, pastries and cake as they have loads of and sugar and are made with refined flour. You can look for multi-grain bread though.

Tip #6: Beat Inflammation And Season Your Food With Spices.

Increase the flavour of bland food with turmeric, garlic, onions, cayenne and ginger. Aside from helping your food taste a lot better, these choices also help in weight reduction.

Tip #7: Stop The Allergies, Food Intolerance And Sensitivities For Good.

You know the food that you are allergic to so it is best to complete take them out of your diet. Disregard the common belief that if you are allergic to a particular food, you should eat it in order to gain immunity. For an Anti-Inflammatory diet, you need to stay away from allergens in order to reduce the inflammation. If you do not know what food causes your allergic reactions, have your doctor give you the Allergy test to find out. Sensitivities are not food-exclusive; any kind of stressor such as taxing activities can aggravate the inflammation.

Tips #8: Increase Your Intake Of Vegetables.

Did you know that when you eat vegetables, it alkalises your body and combats acidity? Inflammation is present when your body is acidic. It is better to include vegetables like cauliflower, broccoli and green leafy vegetables in your menu.

Tip #9: Increase Your Intake Of Gluten-Free Food To Fight Inflammation.

It may help to stick to gluten-free food to prevent inflammation.

Tip #10: Allow Your Body To Run On Glucose In Moderate Amounts.

Eating too much sugar, which your body cannot utilise, can result to inflammation. The Anti-Inflammation Diet requires no sugar at all. If you feel weak, get natural sugar from the fruits that you can eat. Even though you have the thumbs-up to seek sugar from fruits, it does not give you the permission to hoard all sweet-tasting fruits. Glucose will turn into Fructose and can cause inflammation to go haywire. Limit the servings and choose fruits that are low in glycemic index. Examples of low GI fruits are raspberries and blueberries.

Tip #11: Avoid Drive-Through Food And Packaged Ready-To-Eat Food.

Your favourite convenience store food may contain dyes, preservatives, and too much fat calories. Avoid inflammation and allowing these foods to create other ailments such as Alzheimer's disease, ADHD and dementia.

Tip #12: Present Of Fat In Animal Protein Leads To Inflammation. Cut Back Or Take It Out From Your Diet.

Limit intake of fatty meat. If you are suffering from an inflammatory condition, you may eat up to as much as 6 ounces a day. The Anti-Inflammation diet allows meat intake only if the meat were sources from grass-fed animals. The reason here is that the cows and pigs follow a diet that not is heavy with antibiotics. Rather, they eat beans, nuts, and vegetables.

Tip #13: Allow Your Babies To Drink Milk.

Patients who follow the Anti-Inflammation Diet have a reason as to why they follow it. Their bodies are inflamed due to the intake of the wrong kind of food. Milk, however innocent it may be, is a famous inflammatory component. An alternative way of drinking milk is coconut or almond milk.

Tip #14: Avoid Skipping Meals (Even If You Are Not Hungry.)

Do not skip meals since it causes an imbalance to your system. Once you get hungry, the blood sugar levels dip and triggers inflammatory problems. Eat double the volume you need, you raise your insulin levels. It is always better to eat little portions of food throughout the day to prevent or control inflammation.

There are times when you tell yourself that it is okay to skip a meal since you are not hungry. Little did you know, your body is screaming for food! You will feel dizzy, hot-tempered, and weak. All these symptoms are part of an inflamed gut that sends signals to your brains to seek sustenance. You will eventually lose weight with the Anti-Inflammatory Diet since the food is controlled and does not have alarming rebounds.

Tip#15: Aim For Variety

Include as much variety as possible. It is easy to get discouraged when you follow a diet plan. An easy way to ensure that you stay motivated to follow this diet is to have as much variety as possible. As you may be aware, there are several exciting recipes available that can add a lot of variety to your meal plans.

Tip #16: Calorie Intake

Adults are required to consume at least 2,000 to 3,000 calories a day. Women and inactive people need fewer calories. Hence, ensure that your calories are derived in this fashion: 30 percent from fat, 40 percent to 50 percent from carbohydrates and around 20 percent to 30 percent from proteins.

Tip #17: "Fresh" Is The Keyword

Include as much fresh foods in your meal as possible. As such, this diet prescribes the consumption of large quantities of fresh vegetables and fruits. Do not consume processed and packaged foods. Minimise the intake of fast foods as well. You will realise the importance of fibre in fighting inflammation by the end of this book. Hence, it is necessary that you consume foods that are packed with fibre. In other words, consume lots of fruits and vegetables.

Tip #18: Get Your Phytonutrients Right

Phytonutrients play an important role in decreasing your risks of cardiac diseases and also other age related diseases. You can get your required dosage of phytonutrients in the following fashion:

• Include mushrooms, in generous quantities, in your diet.

• When you are choosing your produce, try to go organic as much as possible. This is to avoid the consumption of produce, which are loaded with pesticides.

• Include vegetables and fruits of different colours. Go for tomatoes, berries, leafy greens, oranges, mangoes , etc.

• Include lots of cruciferous vegetables in your diet.

• Go for red wine, if you wish to have alcohol.

• Make sure that you consume lots of soy foods.

Tip #19: Form A Support System

It is easy for any of us to deviate from any diet plan. It is mostly because of the lack of support or the lack of motivation or sometimes both. It is important that you stay on track to reap the maximum benefits of this plan. There are two important things that you need to focus on, before you get started with the diet – goal setting and support system.

It is important that you have goals for your diet plan. Why is goal setting important? Goals add lot more focus to your dieting. Since they are measurable, your goals can also be used to track your progress. Start small, if you are new to goal setting. For instance, if you are not used to dieting before, you can come up with daily goals. Ensure that these goals are in line with the guidelines prescribed by the diet. Once you are used to setting goals for every day, you can extend this principle to setting goals for the week and then the month. When you have such measurable goals in place, you will find it easier to stay on track.

A sound support system is required to keep you motivated at all times. Sometimes, we hesitate to divulge our dieting plans to our friends and family. But, it is highly essential that you have them in the loop about your diet goals. This is because often we tend to deviate from our diet plans out of peer pressure. When you keep your friends and family in the loop, they will seldom pressure you into breaking your diet. Another reason why they should be informed about your diet plans is that you can look to them for motivation, if you feel that you don't have it in you to get on with the diet any further. At such times, their support and motivation can work wonders. Hence, it is highly important that you have a support system in place. Try to get your family members started on this diet too.

Tip #20: Start Slow

If you are new to dieting, you will definitely find it difficult to switch over. It is important that you do not have tall expectations about your resolve in the first few days. It is not humanly possible for anybody to get accustomed to a new diet, without any hassles. There will definitely be some slip ups when you begin. The key is to take it slow and not go hard on yourself. Gradually, switch over to the diet. This way, you will find it easier to adapt. For instance, this diet prescribes the consumption of fresh fruits and vegetables in large quantities. In other words, your fibre intake is considerably increased. If you start consuming so much fibre straight away, it may not sit well with your digestive system and you may face bloating issues as well. So, you need to gradually introduce fibre into your system, if you were previously not in the habit of consuming vegetables and fruits. Take it slow and you will find yourself adapting to this diet easily and in no time.

Tip #21: Reward System

I had mentioned earlier that motivation plays an important role in helping you stay on track. A good way to keep yourself motivated is to have a sound reward system in place. Make sure that these rewards are not food items for they are capable of making us deviate from the diet. Keep a tab on your progress and reward yourself as and when necessary. This is where your goals will come into play. Since they are tangible measures of progress, it will be easier for you to peg your rewards with your goals.

Just like how it is important for you to reward yourself, it is also important that you are not too hard on yourself for any slip ups. Like I mentioned before, it is natural that you deviate from the diet at times. The key is to identify the reasons for these slip ups and come up with measures to ensure that it does not happen again. For instance, if you notice that you are deviating from the diet because of this friend who keeps pushing you to eat out, then it is important that you have a chat with him or her about how significant this diet is to you and what impact it has on your health.

Tip #22: Keep Your Pantry Well Stocked

Many times, people tend to take the easy route and binge on fast food because their pantry is not stocked with the ingredients that they are looking for. So, it is important that you keep your pantry well stocked at all times. When you have all the necessary ingredients in place, you will not have any excuses left to not stick to the diet.

Tip #23: Prepare Your Own Meals

Cook your meals from scratch. This is a good way to ensure that you are sticking to the diet. Try one new recipe every day. This should keep you motivated.

Tip #24: Diet Journal

Maintain a diet journal. Make an entry about every meal that you consume. This will not only help you keep track of your progress but also help you identify the pain points. For instance, if you are finding it difficult to follow a certain guideline prescribed by this diet, you can get in touch with your dietician or doctor and seek their assistance in this regard. Similarly, you will be able to identify if you are allergic to certain foods. Maintaining a diet journal is highly essential if you are already under medication for some other medical condition. If your diet is not working well with your medication, you will be able to identify it by having a glance at your diet journal.

Chapter 4
Aid Inflammation With Natural Remedies

You can help address inflammatory conditions with natural supplements. They contain micronutrients that delay the acceleration of inflammation in the body. Patients with chronic ailments take these supplements to deter pain and prevent other symptoms from settling in. According to medical research, it is a wise decision to include the intake of multivitamins and supplements in the morning since it can help in the overall health of patients.

Here are natural supplements that aid in the reduction of inflammation:

Vitamin D3 – Patients who are deficient in this vitamin should ideally bask longer under the sun since it is rich in vitamin D. However, with the intense heat nowadays, staying out for long hours may lead to melanoma or cancer of the skin. This is where oral supplements come in handy. Research also proves that lathering one's skin with sunscreen reduces the absorption of the vitamin. When you are deficient in this vitamin, chronic inflammatory issues lead to negative levels of bone density and immune system. You may also get your dose of Vitamin D3 from tuna, mackerel, salmon and sardines.

Fish Oil – Omega-3 supplements can also prevent inflammatory issues in the body. Today's modern diet does not have a good supply of this fatty acid that is why ingesting natural fish oil supplements can help. Taking this supplement also promotes bone health as well as regulation of blood sugar. Fish oil can also control asthma, dermatitis, hepatitis and even prostate cancer.

Olive Leaf Extract – This anti-inflammatory supplement has antibacterial and antiviral components that combat a slew of illnesses in the body. It is also an immune enhancer as well as an antioxidant that benefits patients suffering from arthritis. Olive leaf extracts are potent enough to fight inflammation if taken in tea form, capsule or powdered form.

Black Cherry Extract – Inflammation of the joints can seek relief through taking black cherry extract supplements. According to research, black cherries reduce uric acid that causes joint pain and swelling. If taken as a supplement or juice, inflammatory issues may lessen over time.

Weeping Willow Bark – Reduce arthritis inflammation by addressing the deficiency of a body substance called salicylate. It blocks the production of prostaglandins that trigger inflammation. You can compare its anti-inflammatory effect with Aspirin but the advantage of taking a natural supplement such as the Weeping Willow Bark is the risk of bleeding. This natural supplement is available in powdered form or capsules. The usual dose of the supplement is 240 mg/day.

Ginger – These supplements offer pain relief brought about by inflamed joint by reducing biochemical, which promote inflammation. It may take around three months for you to notice the effects those. However, ginger supplements are all natural and do not cause any contraindication with other medications.

Bromelain – Unknown for many, bromelain is an enzyme that resides in pineapples. This enzyme has 100% absorption rate than other enzymes. This means that once it is in the bloodstream, it targets inflammation issues faster than painkillers and inflammatory blockers. You can eat the pineapple fruit everyday but in order to get the right dosage of Bromelain in your system, you need to use a juicer to include the sap from its hard stem.

Devil's Claw Root – Available in capsule-form supplements, this natural remedy for inflammation is one of the favourites of patients challenged with osteoarthritis. Yes, it blocks the pain and can provide temporary relief with the use of topical ointments.

Turmeric Root – Use this natural supplement to ease inflammatory pain. It is also gives relief to digestive problems just like using Ibuprofen. Enjoy it as a tea or in capsule form, the affectivity of Turmeric root supplements comes from curcumin. By inhibiting the activity of its antioxidant property, the Turmeric root enhances immune function and boosts anti-inflammatory components as well.

Guggul Extract – Gum resins found in a native tree in India composes this natural supplement. Guggul has medicinal properties that prevents inflammation aids in weight loss and lowers cholesterol. Take this supplement in capsule form.

Chapter 5
5-Day Anti-Inflammatory Diet Sample Guide

Shown below is a one-week guide for you to understand to achieve your own Anti-Inflammatory Diet, just to give you an idea of how your meal plans would look like. There are no detailed recipes in this chapter.

Notice that you'd still get to eat good food. Just remember that you need to pair your meals only with fresh fruit juice, tea or plain water - ditch sodas.

Day 1

Breakfast: Bacon and Blackberry Buckwheat Pancakes

Lunch: Stir-Fry Chili Pork Tenderloins with Pineapple Chunks

Dinner: Italian Gluten-Free Meatballs

Day 2

Breakfast: Gluten-Free and Dairy-Free Rice Porridge

Lunch: Baked Chicken with a Bowl of Chili Beans and Sweet Potatoes

Dinner: Salmon Salad Sandwich with Cucumber and Yogurt

Day 3

Breakfast: Strawberry French Toasties

Lunch: Shrimp and Kalamata Olives Pasta

Dinner: Zucchini Squash, Carrots and Tomato Soup

Day 4

Breakfast: Orange and Banana Smoothie

Lunch: Seafood Grill with Potato-Garlic Dip

Dinner: Tomato and Corn Chowder with Lime Wedges

Day 5

Breakfast: Scrambled Eggs with Sautéed Vegetables

Lunch: Butter Beans, Brussels sprouts with Rice

Dinner: Kale, Spinach and Broccoli Soup in Coconut Milk

Chapter 6
Foods That Boost The Anti Inflammation Process

If you are planning on adopting the anti-inflammatory diet, you will obviously need to school yourself about the various aspects of the diet. You will need to understand in depth what the diet is about, and this book has so far laid the groundwork for you to be able to do that.

However, there is still one very important piece of information that you have yet to discover, and that is what foods exactly aid the anti-inflammation process. The diet itself is an excellent framework for combating inflammation within your body; however you will need to know what foods exactly you should be eating in order to make that framework work as efficiently as possible.

Hence, what follows is a list of foods that you should eat while you are on this diet. These cover a variety of different food groups and can be considered a more or less comprehensive list of the foods that you should be eating while you are on this diet. Pay attention the details provided about these foods, and try to make sure that your diet consists of foods that are present on this list.

Almonds

The first thing you must understand before you look upon this list of foods that you can eat is that some foods are better at boosting your body's ability to combat inflammation than others. This is why this list is so effective; it helps you to understand what foods are the most efficient at helping your body combat inflammation.

It is a widely known fact that nuts help combat inflammation more than perhaps any other food. However, the hierarchy is present within nuts as well. Some nuts are better at helping you combat inflammation than others.

Near the top of the hierarchy are almonds. They can be eaten as quick snacks between meals and actually make it quite easy for your body to combat inflammation. If you wish to add variety to your daily intake of nuts you can go for other kinds of nuts as well. Good choices include cashew nuts as well as walnuts. Walnuts especially can help you cope with ailments such as rheumatoid arthritis.

Almonds on their own are excellent supplements to your anti-inflammatory diet, but as long as the nuts you are eating are raw you will notice a decrease in inflammation in your body.

Apple Cider Vinegar

The recent boom in fad diets and the emergence of healthcare as a veritable subculture has led to a number of foods being advertised as super foods. These foods are supposedly extremely dense in nutrients and can cure a variety of ailments. As it turns out, few of these foods are actually as healthy as they are advertised.

However, one exception to this rule is apple cider vinegar. This particular type of vinegar is compatible with the vast majority of diets from detox to ketogenic. However, the diet that it is, perhaps, most compatible with is in fact the one you are reading about right now!

Yes, the nutrients present within apple cider vinegar are very specifically able to target inflammation within your body, which makes this the perfect dressing for that salad you are planning to have for lunch. If you do not like the way your apple cider vinegar tastes with dressing, you can try taking a tablespoon before your meal to increase your appetite.

However you choose to consume it, just remember to make it an integral part of your diet. Doing so will vastly decrease the amount of inflammation in your joints especially.

Apricots

As you read in the section about almonds, there is a hierarchy of food and several sub hierarchies within specific food groups as well. As far as fruits go, there are several out there that can be considered contenders for the top spot. One of the most important fruits that you can consume while you are on your anti inflammation diet is, without a doubt, apricot.

You might know by now that some of the most important nutrients that you can consume while you are trying to combat chronic inflammation within your body are phytochemicals. Apricots contain a very specific phytochemical called quercetin that can be instrumental for your body in its struggle against chronic inflammation.

Thus, it is very important that you incorporate apricots into your diet in order to bring the level of chronic inflammation way down. A great way to do so is to add apricots to your salads. Apricot is one of the fruits that actually go really well with salads, and a somewhat unorthodox but truly delicious combination that you can try is apricot and spinach. Add a little dressing in the form of extra virgin olive oil and you will have for yourself a delicious and incredibly healthy lunch.

Asparagus

It can be argued that apple cider vinegar is not really a food, which means that it can't really be called a superfood simply because it cannot be eaten on its own. Rather, apple cider vinegar has to be added to your recipes as a dressing or something similar. It cannot be the main ingredient in your meal.

However, asparagus is definitely a food, and as it turns out it is actually on the most effective super foods that you could possibly eat. It is particularly effective against inflammation, so if you are feeling as though your inflammation is not going down you can add asparagus to your meals to help speed the process up.

Asparagus is one of the most effective vegetables that you can possibly eat as far as the anti-inflammatory diet goes. It is important to distinguish between vegetables that don't aid your diet and vegetables that do, and since asparagus is one of the latter you should really eat it as often as possible.

The versatility of asparagus allows you to eat it on the side of your main meal as well as on its own.

Avocado

One thing that prevents the asparagus from the being the best vegetable that it can possibly be is that it does not taste all that great. Us humans are put off by things that do not fulfil our base desires, which means that no matter how healthy the asparagus is, we are probably not going to want to eat it all that much simply because it doesn't taste that great.

However, the problem is solved somewhat if we look at the avocado. The avocado has the distinction of tasting excellent, which means that we are more likely to eat it. It doesn't hurt that it is also jam packed with nutrients that can greatly aid our body in its fight against inflammation.

It is also a very versatile food because it aids in fat loss as well as it replaces the unhealthy saturated fats that we tend to consume with fats that are actually very good for you.

Incorporating avocados into your diet is actually quite easy. Just add them to your salads and you will find that they will taste better and will be a lot better for your health as well.

Basil

One thing that this list has missed out on so far is seasoning. Sometimes you just need something to add some true flavour to the food that you are eating. After all, if we do not add variety to our meals it is going to be extremely difficult for us to follow this diet at all.

Hence, it is very important for us to incorporate spices into our meals. However, there are certain spices that you can favour simply due to the fact that they contain nutrients and chemicals that will aid you in your quest to decrease the inflammation in your body.

One of the best spices that you can use is basil. The nutrients contained within basil actually specifically reduce chronic inflammation, making it an excellent herb for you to add to your meals. Rosemary and parsley are also excellent ways to add flavour to your food while simultaneously making it easier for your body to reduce its chronic inflammation.

Simply add a dash of each herb, find a mixture that suits you, to your meals and you will find that they will taste a lot better. Over time you will feel the swelling of your joints recede as well!

Bell Peppers

Some foods are simply gifts from a higher being, or at least they seem that way. This is mostly due to the fact that these foods are both delicious and incredibly good for you.

Some good examples of such foods are bell peppers. Bell peppers are a great addition to your meals, and are actually an integral part of westernised Chinese cuisine, and can even be used in salads to add distinct peppery flavour without upping the spiciness quotient all that much.

Apart from being utterly delicious, bell peppers are also excellent sources of a specific form of antioxidant called flavonoids. Flavonoids are actually what make bell peppers so good at making the anti-inflammatory diet more efficient. You are made more able to fight inflammation when your body has been purged of certain toxins.

One thing that you must make sure of while eating bell peppers is that you need to incorporate all of the different colours available. Each colour has a different type of flavonoids, and each of these types is very important for your overall diet. Incorporate them into your salads, and try to get each colour in at the same time. Not only will your food become really healthy, it will look really pretty too!

Black Beans

Beans are also a very important part of your anti-inflammatory diet for slightly more practical reasons. They offer your body a very healthy source of an absolutely essential nutrient: protein.

The problem with protein is that most people think that they can only get it from meat. Meat is not all that compatible with the anti-inflammatory diet as you already know. This means that beans provide a very useful alternative to meat as far as acquiring your daily required dose of protein goes.

Beans are also great at boosting the anti-inflammatory process, and a lot of restaurants have started offering them as side dishes. This means that you can substitute unhealthy side dishes such as French fries or mashed potatoes with a healthier alternative that is more likely to help you improve your anti-inflammatory diet.

Black beans are preferable simply because it is easier to find them. Incorporate them into your salads in order to improve the protein quantity of your daily meals. Remember that protein is one of the most important nutrients out there, so stocking up on it will only do your body good.

Blueberries

If there is one thing that this list has been missing, it is something sweet to chew on. As has been said several times before, we are the kind of people that would eat something that is terribly bad for us as long as it tastes good before we eat something that is really very good for us simply because this healthy food happens to taste bad.

Sweet, healthy foods are actually very common. They are called fruit! Apricots are sweet but they are more for regular meals and can't substitute your snacks. For that, you can use blueberries instead!

In fact, practically any berry would do, blueberries are just a better option because they taste the best and contain the most nutrients that would improve your body's struggle against inflammation.

Berries are an excellent addition to your anti-inflammatory diet because they possess both antioxidants as well as phytonutrients. This combination of nutrients makes it really easy for your body to bring down the chronic inflammation in your joints.

You can make smoothies out of them, use them in fruit salads or just eat a bunch of them as a snack. Just try to incorporate berries into your diet as much as possible.

Bok Choy

Bok Choy is basically a slightly odd looking cauliflower. The similarity is due to the fact that it is a cruciferous vegetable much like broccoli and cauliflower but the similarities end there simply because bok choy is far better for your health than either of these vegetables.

In fact, bok choy is arguably one of the healthiest vegetables in the world. It is an excellent source of beta carotene as well as vitamin A and is chock full of phytonutrients that can boost your body's ability to fight chronic inflammation.

However, you are probably not eating this vegetable all that often. This probably because you simply do not think of it all that much, that when you go out shopping for vegetables you end up getting broccoli instead. While all cruciferous vegetables are important in your overall diet, you will find that bok choy is perhaps better at specifically fighting inflammation than all of the rest, and can certainly help broccoli to do the wonderful job that it is already doing.

You can consume this vegetable in a variety of ways, but instead of just putting it into a salad try to be a little different and stir fry it with some other vegetables and some soy sauce.

Broccoli

Just because bok choy has some excellent nutrients that help tackle inflammation, broccoli is still probably one of the most important vegetables that you can consume at least as far as overall health is concerned.

In order to fight inflammation, it is very important that you make your overall body healthy. Just eating foods that fight inflammation will probably result in your body not having all that much energy left to take care of all of the other functions that are so important.

Broccoli helps with everything that bok choy can't. It is full of protein, one of the only vegetables that can give you a decent amount of the nutrient, has more vitamin C than even oranges, and can help to treat and even prevent certain diseases.

Overall, broccoli is an absolute must have in your anti inflammation diet. Buy it organic and fresh wherever possible and incorporate it into your diet. If you combine bok choy and broccoli as efficiently as they are meant to be together, you will soon find that your inflammation has begun to go down and you are not as tired and lazy as you used to be.

Brussels Sprouts

As far as the world of vegetables is concerned, Brussels sprouts don't have a particularly good reputation. This is for a variety of reasons, one of these reasons being that they simply don't taste good. Another, somewhat silly, reason is that Brussels sprouts actually cause gassiness. Flatulence is frowned upon in society, which means that foods that encourage the situation are avoided as much as possible.

However, Brussels sprouts actually don't deserve their bad reputation. They may not taste all that great, but combined with the right spices and cooking style they can actually form a tasty part of your meals. Additionally, Brussels sprouts certainly do not deserve their reputation for giving people gas. That only happens when you pair them with the wrong kind of food and eat too much of them at the same time.

Brussels sprouts can actually be a very important part of your anti-inflammatory diet simply because the specific set of nutrients that they contain can help reduce inflammation in joints. This makes this vegetable very useful especially for people who are suffering from arthritis.

Buckwheat

Out of all of the foods that you have seen so far on this list, perhaps none was as consumed as buckwheat. It is so rarely consumed because it is not easily available, and people tend to go for regular wheat instead.

However, buckwheat is very commonly eaten in Japan in the form of noodles. As it turns out, inflammation in Japanese people is actually quite low, and it is no coincidence that a low prevalence of chronic inflammation occurs in a place where the consumption of buckwheat is so high because buckwheat, in whatever form it is eaten, is one of the best foods in the world as far as reducing inflammation goes.

There are several ways to incorporate buckwheat, and once you start doing so you will actually learn the nutty taste of buckwheat is actually a great addition to any dish. This nutty taste goes very well with pancakes, so if you are thinking of incorporating buckwheat into your diet the best way to do so would be to start eating buckwheat pancakes. They are absolutely delicious and will add a great amount of nutrients to your diet. You can also give buckwheat noodles a try. The flavour is different but many people state that it is quite enjoyable.

Cabbage

Cabbage is a great vegetable, but if you opt for red cabbage you will be receiving the additional benefit of being able to consume anthocyanin. Anthocyanin's are an extremely important part of your anti-inflammatory diet because they are able to reduce the excess blood flow to the swollen joints and are particularly effective at reducing joint pain.

However, this does not mean that other types of cabbage should not be incorporated into your diet. If you are unable to find red cabbage, just incorporate regular cabbage into your diet and you will begin to see some great benefits straight away. This is because cabbages cruciferous vegetables and contain a lot of nutrients that help bring inflammation down.

The best way to consume cabbage is in the form of soup. You can add spices to make it taste better and the cabbage itself becomes softer and easier to digest. You can make cabbage soup in bulk and eat it for lunch every other day! Just remember to eat some brown bread with it as well so that you are getting your daily requirement of carbohydrates and fibre in as well.

Cantaloupe

The great thing about fruits is that they give you so many extraordinary health benefits, benefits that truly cannot be derived from multivitamin pills or anything of that sort, while at the same time tasting so great. Indeed, once you have weaned yourself off your sugar addiction you will find that there is no dessert or snack that is superior to fruit

In the hierarchy of fruit, there are very few fruits that manage to rank higher than cantaloupe. This is simply because cantaloupe is a near perfect mixture of health and taste! They are jam packed with phytonutrients and are also full of vitamin A and C as well!

This means that cantaloupes are able to combat inflammation whilst simultaneously detoxifying your body as well. This means that while the phytonutrients reduce the inflammation, the process of detoxification puts your body in a position to handle the chronic disease that you are suffering from on its own.

The importance of cantaloupes is greatly increased by the fact that they taste so great. Cantaloupes make a handy dessert and can even be used as a midday snack. You can switch between berries and cantaloupes to add a little variety to your diet!

Carrots

Vegetables are generally considered to be healthy foods to eat. However, carrots are those vegetables that are perhaps the most widely praised in health circles because they are full to the brim with several different kinds of nutrients which can help your body to fight inflammation.

Carrots are one of the most popular sources of beta carotene in the world. Although the similarity between carrot and carotene is somewhat unintentional, carrots are in fact one of the best ways that you can get your daily dose of the essential nutrients. Carrots are also very important sources of vitamin A that can help to remove toxins from your body that might be causing inflammation.

There are many ways to incorporate carrots into your diet. Salads are the obvious choice, but you can also use carrots dipped in hummus as an excellent midday snack or as an appetiser before your main meal. However, the best way to eat your carrots is, perhaps, in the form of a juice. This is because it is often difficult to chew carrots enough to release enough of the precious nutrients it holds. Drinking carrot juice allows you to get these nutrients while simultaneously giving your jaw a bit of a rest.

Cauliflower

Although not as versatile as broccoli or as specifically suited to the anti-inflammatory processes as bok choy, cauliflower is a cruciferous vegetable, and all cruciferous vegetables play an important role in the anti-inflammation process. However, cauliflower has one up over its more flamboyant cousins in the fact that it contains a nutrient that is essential for well-maintained health but has gained a reputation for being notoriously elusive: vitamin K.

Since vitamin K is so difficult to find, the fact that cauliflower has it in spades is enough to justify its presence in your diet. However, cauliflower also happens to be an excellent source of vitamin C, which means that you need to stock up on this vegetable if you want your body to be healthy enough to fight inflammation.

Its antioxidants and anti-inflammatory properties make cauliflower an important part of any anti-inflammatory diet worth its sort. It does not taste that great raw, so try adding it to a stir fry of various cruciferous vegetables. This will give the vegetables a great oriental flavour and will help you to keep your daily dose of phytonutrients up.

Celery

Celery has a reputation for being diet food. This might be because it has a reputation for not tasting very good and is very low in calories. However, celery's reputation, much like the reputation of other vegetables in this list, is not all that accurate.

It is true that celery is very low in calories, but it is chock full of nutrients as well. This means that you can eat quite a bit of it to get your daily dose of nutrients in before hitting your maximum limit of daily caloric intake. However, it does not actually taste all that bad

Some people may be put off by celery's unique and somewhat spicy taste or it's rather stringy texture, but these people simply don't know how to eat celery properly. Celery on its own does not taste that great, but that does not mean that you can't incorporate it successfully into your diet.

The best way to eat celery is, believe it or not, as a snack. Take a stick of celery, smear it with some peanut butter and add raisins. You now have a snack that is crunchy, salty and sweet and is full of nutrients! Incorporating celery into your diet is a great way to boost your body's fight against inflammation due to its anti-inflammatory properties.

Chicken

It is a widely accepted fat that meat is not a very good part of any anti-inflammatory diet. This is because meat tends to cause inflammation rather than remove it, and such foods absolutely have to be cut out of your diet if you want to bring the inflammation in your joints down.

However, a major problem with cutting meat out of diets completely is that most people are simply unable to do it. We have become so used to eating meat as a part of our daily meals that we would abandon any diet that cuts these meats out.

Chicken, and other white meats, are the happy medium in this scenario because they do not have as many inflammatory chemicals as red meats do. This means that you can incorporate chicken and other white meat into your diet without worrying too much about inflaming your joints.

However, it is highly recommended that you try to cut meat out of your diet completely. Doing so might actually help you a lot more in the long run and is definitely worth a try.

Cinnamon

Spices are an important part of any diet, because without spices we might actually abandon our diet a lot earlier simply because the food is too bland. However, as has been stated before, some spices are a lot more beneficial for you during this diet than others, and cinnamon is one of them.

Cinnamon has a reputation for being a cure for a wide variety of chronic diseases. While it is uncertain whether cinnamon truly is the all-purpose cure that some people make it out to be, the spice has been proven to have a positive effect on inflammation. This is due to the fact that its unique set of nutrients actually helps the body to reduce swelling of joints in particular.

There are several ways in which you can incorporate cinnamon into your diet. Most people just sprinkle a bit of cinnamon into the food that they are cooking. My personal favourite is to add cinnamon to my tea when I drink it. I simply add a couple of sticks of cinnamon per cup of tea while the water is boiling. This makes the tea taste better and helps to reduce inflammation as well!

Cucumber

Cucumber is usually seen as a refreshing vegetable that can help refresh you during the summer. It is an excellent source of refreshment to be sure, but it is hardly being used to its full potential if this is all that it is being used for.

Cucumber is not just ultra-hydrating; it is full of extremely important antioxidants as well. The overall combinations of nutrients that are present within a cucumber are actually conducive to two specific processes that end up helping each other out in the long run. These two processes are detoxification and a reduction in inflammation.

Eating cucumbers will allow you to use its specific nutrients to reduce inflammation whilst simultaneously removing harmful toxins from your body that would make it difficult for your body to heal itself while in the throes of chronic inflammation.

Cucumbers can be incorporated into your salads to make them a lot fresher and healthier, but they can also be drunk in the form of a smoothie. A somewhat underrated method of consuming cucumbers is in the form of cucumber soup. If you live in a hot climate, cucumber soup can be used to greatly refresh you during the heat of the afternoon.

Curry Powder

Hindu culture is ancient and it is fully of many hidden remedies for the vast majority of modern ailments. Hence, it is no surprise that curry powder, an ingredient used extensively in Indian cuisine, is the source of so many anti-inflammatory properties.

Indian culture has a very low prevalence of chronic inflammatory disease and it is simply because they use curry powder, an ingredient that is full of anti-inflammatory properties, in the vast majority of dishes that are popular within said culture. There is always science to be found behind these correlations.

Incorporating curry into your diet is easy, simply start cooking curries! Indian curries are often vegetarian based as well, which means that you can turn the majority of your main meals into Indian dishes and still follow your anti-inflammatory diet to a great degree of accuracy.

Just remember to keep your consumption of fruits up, and keep in mind that fresh vegetables are far healthier than cooked ones, so make sure that you don't rely on Indian curries to provide you with your daily intake of vegetables. Try having salads with your curries to keep things interesting and wholesome!

Dark Chocolate

This entry is perhaps going to perk up a few interested ears. Dark chocolate is a world renowned delicacy, and is often claimed by purists to be the only form of chocolate that is worth consuming, since milk chocolate is filled with nothing but sugar anyway.

Dark chocolate is not just a tasty treat; it is an excellent way to reduce inflammation as well and can actually become a very useful and important part of your anti-inflammatory diet. It is full of antioxidants and can actually help detoxify your body to some extent as well, which is additional to its enormous quantity of phytonutrients of course.

Dark chocolate can be used as a treat that you can consume between meals, but don't go overboard because it's still not exactly good for you. Your snacks should mostly consist of berries and fruit, dark chocolate can be used sparingly to give yourself the occasional treat for doing such a great job.

However, make absolutely sure that you avoid milk chocolate like the plague. Milk chocolate is full of processed sugar that has inflammatory properties. Eating milk chocolate will greatly reduce the efficacy of your anti-inflammatory diet.

Eggs

This may seem like a somewhat odd entry in a list that encourages wholesome foods, but that is only because the recent crop of fad diets has, for some reason, vilified eggs as some kind of evil foods that are chock full of cholesterol. While it is true that egg yolks have cholesterol, these yolks can be removed, the cholesterol isn't all that harmful anyway and, most importantly, you aren't looking to lose weight in this diet, you are looking to reduce the inflammation in your body.

All you need to make sure of is that the eggs you purchase have added omega-3 fatty acids in them. This is because omega-3 is actually a great source of anti-inflammatory nutrients that can help your body to fight the chronic inflammations that are plaguing it.

Eggs are important because, since you can't eat all that much meat, they can serve as an excellent substitute to get your daily supply of protein in. Eat them on their own or as part of other dishes, just make sure that you don't eat them every day and you will be good to go. Try to mix your daily protein intake up between eggs and legumes as well as vegetable sources.

Extra Virgin Olive Oil

Perhaps as a result of the vast majority of turn of the century cooking shows referring to it as the ultimate dressing and cooking oil, extra virgin olive oil has become sensationally popular. This is also due to the fact that it EVOO, as it is so often called, is also the healthiest cooking oil there is, as it has the lowest amount of cholesterol and is very low in calories.

Extra virgin olive oil is very important in your diet, and it might just turn out to be the single most important component in your quest to reduce the chronic inflammation that is plaguing your body. This is because its anti-inflammatory properties are fantastic, to the point where it is almost as effective as drugs that are designed to treat inflammation without possessing any of the side effects.

You can use EVOO in a variety of ways. It can, and should, become your go to cooking oil, it is a great dressing for salads because it is light in both flavour and texture and can just be used to add some texture to dishes that are a little too dry.

Fennel

Fennel is another food that is wildly popular in Hindu culture and contributes greatly to the extremely low prevalence of chronic inflammation in that part of the world.

The concentration of phytonutrients and antioxidants in fennel is superior to perhaps any other food, for the tiny little seed that is fennel actually contains almost as many nutrients as many larger alternatives. It is so full of phytonutrients and antioxidants that incorporating fennel into your diet can actually boost the amount of anti-inflammatory nutrients you are eating by a significant amount even if the amount of fennel you are incorporating is somewhat low.

Fennel can be eaten in a variety of ways. As an herb it can incorporated into your recipes and it can even be used to spice up your alcoholic drinks if you partake in that sort of thing. However, perhaps the most underrated use for fennel is as a mouth freshener. Fennel is somewhat spicy on the outside and on the inside it is incredibly sweet. The fragrance of it floods your mouth to the point where you can hide the smell of alcohol with it! It's no wonder that fennel is commonly eaten on its own in countries such as India and Pakistan.

Flaxseed

When the recent health craze erupted, there were several foods that were touted as being superior to all others as far as health and weight loss was concerned. One of these foods was flaxseeds, and flax seeds were one of the rare foods that were part of this health craze that were actually beneficial for your health.

Flaxseeds contain very specific nutrients in the form of lignans and alpha-Linoleic acids. These nutrients combat inflammation specifically, to the point where it is speculated that your body specifically absorbs these nutrients for no other purpose than to combat inflammation. It also helps that flaxseeds are very important source of omega-3 fatty acids, which as you already know are a very important part of your overall anti-inflammatory diet.

Incorporating flaxseed into your diet is also extremely easy. All you really need to do is sprinkle the seed over any food that you are eating. The seeds themselves have little to no flavour, which means that you can incorporate them into your salads to greatly boost the nutritional content without having to worry about how the addition will end up affecting the taste of your lunch.

Garlic

Many people will rejoice to know that garlic is in this list, simply because garlic is such a delicious vegetable to have in your diet. It is a staple in Italian culture, but is also very prevalent in Indian culture as well. It is no wonder that Indian people have such a low rate of inflammatory disease considering that their diets incorporate so many different foods that contain such strong anti-inflammatory properties!

In fact, if there is one thing health gurus, doctors and even people who have actually suffered from chronic inflammation can agree on, it's that garlic is perhaps one of the most important and effective foods that you can possibly eat while you are on your anti-inflammatory diet. In fact, many doctors prescribe pills with ingredients derived from garlic to combat inflammation.

The best way to consume garlic is in a paste or to slice it up before you add it to your food. Garlic has a lot of locked nutrients which means that slicing the vegetable before you consume it will allow you to get to all of those hidden nutrients a lot more easily than if you were to add the entire clove of garlic whole.

Ginger

In Indian culture, there is a golden rule that most chefs follow and that is that garlic and ginger always go together. If you need proof that a food definitely has anti-inflammatory properties, all you need to do is find out if it is regularly eaten in Indian culture. If it is, as is the case with both garlic and ginger, you can rest assured that this food will have a lot to give you as far as anti-inflammatory diets are concerned.

Ginger contains a nutrient known as gingerols, which actually is very beneficial for people who are suffering from chronic inflammation. You can add ginger to your tea (just remember not to add milk along with it!) or stir fry it along with other vegetables to add flavor but the best way to incorporate ginger into your diet is to mash it into a paste, mix it up with mashed up garlic and use the combined paste to cook your curries.

This will add a unique and authentic flavor to your curries while simultaneously greatly boosting the anti-inflammatory properties of the food that you are eating. You can even add this paste to your stir fries instead of using whole ginger or garlic!

Grapefruit

Grapefruit has long been considered a healthy fruit and for good reason. It is one of the few fruits that are genuinely low in sugar, which means that you can enjoy the myriad health benefits that grapefruit has to offer without worrying about the various health implications that come with eating massive amounts of sugar.

Some people are put off at first by the taste of grapefruit, but if you stick with it you will find that not all the tasty things in life are sweet. Grapefruits unique tangy and pungent combination is a gift to your taste buds; all you really need to do is get used to the taste in the first place.

It is important that you incorporate grapefruit into your diet because it contains a lot of antioxidants that can help your anti inflammation diet become a lot more efficient.

You can incorporate grapefruit into your diet by turning it into a smoothie or by using it in a salad but I highly recommend that you do not try to mask its flavor. Eat it as it is and learn to appreciate its unique taste!

Green tea

There is nothing more relaxing than a beverage at the end of a long day of work. Water sometimes just doesn't cut it, sometimes you need something that you can just lay back and sip without a care in the world. It is a great way to unwind and, as it turns it, if the drink in question is tea than you are actually doing your body a huge favor!

Tea is full of antioxidants, and green tea especially is full of flavonoids. You will have heard of them in this list by now, and rightly so because flavonoids are extremely important tools that can help your body reduce inflammation. This means that tea is actually a very important part of your anti-inflammatory diet, which goes nicely with the fact that it is a very relaxing drink as well.

Try out different herbal tea mixes to spice things up, just make sure that you are consuming tea that has flavonoids in it. Additionally, you can add ginger to your tea to add a bit of flavor, you will be surprised at just how good strong black tea flavored with ginger and honey can taste!

Hot Sauce

If you have not already been surprised by the entries that are present within this list, you are certainly going to be surprised by the presence of hot sauce. This is probably because you associate hot sauce with inflammation, since, logically, hot sauce is flaming hot!

Inflammation actually has nothing to do with the spiciness of the food that you are eating. Rather, it has more to do with how your body reacts to this food. Unless the inflammation that you are experiencing is heartburn, in which case you should avoid this particular entry in this list, you can definitely incorporate hot sauce into your daily meals! The only other case in which you should avoid hot sauce is you have an upset stomach, as hot sauce will only exacerbate your discomfort.

This is because the very thing that makes hot sauce taste so spicy, a chemical called capsaicin, is an important source of antioxidants. This is what gives bell peppers their antioxidant properties as well! The purpose of this entry is to provide you with an alternative whereby you can spice up and add variety to the foods that you are eating. After all, nobody likes a boring diet!

Kale

This entry might have you rolling your eyes simply because you will have heard pretty much every single "health expert" worth his or her salt tell you that kale is a superfood and it should be incorporated into your diet. This is actually true, kale is one of the few foods that the recent health craze forced into the spotlight that has actual value in our diets. It is also important to mention kale because most people don't take it seriously, and if you are serious about your anti-inflammatory diet you will actually try as hard as you can to incorporate kale into it!

Kale is one of the densest sources of nutrients in the world, from Vitamin C to Vitamin A, and it is also an excellent source of fiber to boot. Kale is actually so effective in it anti-inflammatory properties that it has, in some cases, been known to not just stop the spreading of inflammation in your body, but to reverse it completely! This means that if you incorporate kale into your diet you will not just be keeping your inflammation in check; you might end up curing it altogether!

Kelp

Most people never eat kelp because, after all, it's seaweed! It was never thought of as a food, at least as far as American diets are concerned, but in other cultures it is far more commonly eaten and these cultures happen to have a far lower rate of chronic inflammatory disease as well.

Kelp is an absolutely essential part of your anti-inflammatory diet for several reasons. First and foremost, kelp is able to keep your internal body on the alkaline side of things. You will know by now that an acidic internal chemical composition is actually one of the major causes of inflammation, particularly when the inflammation in question is heartburn.

Kelp also possesses a decent amount of iodine as well, which helps to further balance out your body's internal PH levels and keep your inflammation in check. Kelp also contains something called "fucoidan" which is actually unique to this particular type of food. Fucoidan contains enormous anti-inflammatory properties, so incorporating it into your diet is actually a great way to boost the efficacy of your anti-inflammatory diet.

Although it is a bit tricky to find, kelp is well worth the effort.

Kiwi

If you are well versed in the world of anti-inflammatory foods you might find the addition of kiwi fruit a bit odd in this list. This is because kiwi is not exactly an anti-inflammatory fruit. It has some anti-inflammatory properties but on the whole there are other fruits out there that have much more potent anti-inflammatory properties than kiwi fruit.

However, you need to keep in mind that this list is a comprehensive list of the foods that you can eat while you are on your anti-inflammatory diet. You should not have to have any foods that are not on this list, and so kiwifruit has been added because it has some anti inflammatory properties, is a good source of nutrition and is overall a very tasty fruit that would add variety to your diet and allow you to keep things entertaining instead of sticking with the same old fruit over and over again.

You can eat kiwi fruit on its own, which I would recommend since it tastes fantastic, but you can also mix it up in a fruit salad or incorporate it into a smoothie. Use it to break the monotony of the same old fruits over and over again.

Lemons

Lemons, along with limes, might be some of the most useful things that are on this list. This is because lemons are extremely healthy, full of antioxidants as they are, but they are also useful because of their flavor. You would be hard pressed to find a fruit that is as tangy and sour as the lemon, which makes the juice of this fruit an excellent dressing for salads. In fact, you can use the juice as the sole dressing of your salad and not have to worry about the calories that come with regular dressings.

Lemons also help by cleansing the body of toxins and, ironically, help to increase the alkalinity of your internal chemical composition. This may come as a surprise to your as lemons are acidic by nature, but your body reacts to the presence of lemon juice in your digestive tract by releasing bracing chemicals that boost your internal alkalinity disproportionate to the amount of lemon juice you have consumed.

Use lemons and limes to add a tangy flavor to your meals. You would be doing yourself a favor by adding flavor in such a natural way!

Lentils

You might remember the rule of thumb that was stated earlier about whether food is genuinely helpful to anti-inflammatory diets or not. This rule stated that if a food was part of Indian cuisine, there was a strong chance that it would be enormously beneficial to your anti-inflammatory diet.

Lentils are one of these foods that form an enormous part of Indian cuisine, and contribute greatly to the low prevalence of chronic inflammatory disease within that geographical region. This is because lentils contain anti-inflammatory properties such as phytonutrients.

Lentils are also extremely important because they can be used to help you reach your daily required dose of protein to help keep your body strong enough to keep chronic inflammation at bay. You can use lentils when you don't want to use eggs or if you don't like feeling broccoli on any particular day (for which I won't blame you).

Lentils are great way to add thickness and texture to soup, and boiled and with a bit of salt and lemon can prove to be a great snack that will help you to keep up your blood sugar levels between meals. They are great for diabetics too since they are slow digesting carbohydrates that won't release a flood of sugar into your bloodstream!

Oats

You might be a little lost as far as breakfast is concerned if you are following this diet and I don't blame you. None of the foods here really work with breakfast. You'll just be having fruits or the occasional egg, which is the only real breakfast food that is on this list unless you make buckwheat pancakes.

However, you will notice that this section is about oats. Oats are an excellent breakfast food, and were actually the origin of what breakfast cereals are today! You can incorporate this food into your breakfast and start your day with its important anti-inflammatory properties.

A great way to eat oats is to mix them up with milk and honey and heat up the whole bowl. You can add chia seeds for extra nutritional value or blueberries or any other kinds of berries both for the aforementioned nutritional value and for the fact that the combination is going to taste really good. Having a breakfast like this will give you enough energy to get through a busy day of work and you might not even be hungry for lunch!

Onions

Onions are an excellent vegetable. They are a staple vegetable in Pakistani and Indian cultures, which will prove to you that onion has in it some truly remarkable anti-inflammatory properties. It doesn't hurt that the incredible sharp taste of this vegetable is a great way to spice up your salads and make them more exciting!

Onion is also a great source of quercetin, and is the only the second food on this list so far that has this vital nutrient. Quercetin is absolutely essential in your anti-inflammatory diet, being one of the few nutrients that can be considered as "anti-inflammatory" by nature.

I have included onions in this list not just because they taste great and are a great source of quercetin but because they are extremely cheap too. A lot of the foods on this list are expensive, kelp for example, and health should not be something that only the wealthy can afford. Eating onions is a way to incorporate healthy vegetables into your diet without hurting your wallet too much. It doesn't hurt that they are available all year long either, which means that you can make them a constant in your every changing diet.

Oranges

You might have been wondering when oranges was going to turn up in this list. It was a shoo-in, but the only problem was that this list is alphabetically ordered! Otherwise oranges are some of the most important fruits that you could possibly consume while you are on your diet.

This is because they are extremely important sources of vitamin C as well as antioxidants. Vitamin C is famous for being good for your joints, which means that if the chronic inflammation that you are suffering from is arthritis then you can incorporate oranges into your diet and enjoy the benefits.

The best way to incorporate oranges into your diet is to eat them for breakfast. Try not to overload on the acidic fruits, choose between one of them so as not to make your internal chemical composition overly acidic, but choose oranges as much as you can because they are simply the best citric fruits that you can possibly eat.

Orange juice is also a great beverage that you can use to accompany meals. Its strong flavor can accentuate certain qualities in your food, much like wine or beer does!

Papaya

Here we have another fruit that is perhaps not as popular as it should be, at least in the US. Papaya is an excellent fruit because it is so chock full of all of the nutrients that your body needs to deal with your chronic inflammatory diseases. In fact, papaya contains a lot of phytonutrients that are not present in other fruits, which makes this particular fruit an especially important part of your anti-inflammatory diet.

One thing that you need to understand about phytonutrients is that there is a wide variety of them. This means that a lot of these fruits that are on this list don't contain some of the phytonutrients that others would contain. You can be sure that absolutely no fruit contains the specific phytonutrients that papaya contains.

Hence, if you want to get a balanced amount of phytonutrients into your system, thereby greatly improving the efficacy of your anti-inflammatory diet, you need to eat as many of the different fruits in this list as possible. However, it is highly recommended that you make papaya an indispensable part of your diet. As has been said twice already, papaya has nutrients that no other fruit does, and these nutrients can really help your body fight inflammation.

Pineapple

Kiwi was added in this list because it tastes good and doesn't do your body any harm. Pineapple has been added to this list because it tastes good and is a veritable powerhouse of anti-inflammatory properties.

There are many foods like pineapple out there, food that tastes amazing and is actually very food for your anti inflammatory diet. Pineapple is one of them, and is one of the most important fruits that you can possibly incorporate into your diet, but the truly great thing about pineapple is its taste.

The vast majority of fruits that you will have seen in this list have been acidic. Pineapple is one of the few that is genuinely sweet without being tangy at all. In fact, pineapple is so sweet that it can be considered a delicacy in and of itself. However, if you are diabetic or are looking to lose weight, be careful with the portion sizes that you consume.

Experiment with portion sizes and consult a doctor before you start consuming pineapple if you are diabetic. Remember, diabetes is a disease too and your diet should reflect the fact that you have this disease.

Pumpkin

Pumpkin is one of the most versatile vegetables in this comprehensive list of the foods that you can eat while you are following the anti inflammatory diet. This is because there are so many ways in which it can be eaten. You can roast its flesh, turn it into a soup, even pumpkin seeds are a great source of nutrition and can be used as a light snack to keep yourself going between meals.

Like most of the other foods in this list, pumpkins contain phytochemicals that help your body to keep inflammation down. However, it is also important to note that this vegetable is here because you can do so much with it. A lot of the foods in this list have been added so that you can add some variety to the meals that you are eating. Pumpkins are great way to add said variety.

Pumpkins are also very useful because they are so filling. You can eat a little bit of pumpkin and be full for a long time. Small meals are an important part of the anti-inflammatory diet because they help your body focus on fighting inflammation rather than digesting the food that you have eaten.

Quinoa

Quinoa is a wonder food in truth, unlike the vast majority of foods that have become massively popular after the recent health craze that the world has gone through. Quinoa is an amazing source of fiber as well as protein, but what really sets this food apart is the fact that it possesses such a unique mix of vitamins and minerals. In fact, no other food contains the specific mixture of vitamins and minerals that quinoa contains, which means that you really should try as hard as you can to incorporate this food into your anti-inflammatory diet.

Quinoa's unique mix of nutrients aside, this food is also very filling. You will remember from the previous entry in this list that a big part of the anti inflammatory diet is helping your body focus on the healing process without bogging it down with excessive digestion. You boost its anti-inflammatory properties and give it as little else to do as possible so that it can focus. One of the most important things that quinoa does is that it bulks up your meals and helps them become more filling so that you don't have to eat as much.

Red wine

Perhaps no food, or drink rather, in this entire list will give people as much joy as red wine. We love to drink, this is a fact. It helps us socialize and is just plain fun. As it turns out, drinking can be good for you, as long as the drink that you are consuming is wine.

While it is highly recommended that you avoid alcohol as it can severely exacerbate the inflammation that you are suffering from, red wine happens to possess flavonoids that help to create a balance. This means that red wine is not as bad for you as other alcoholic drinks are and can be drunk in moderation while you are on your anti-inflammatory diet.

However, keep in mind that beer and spirits are not recommended at all. They do not contain any of the restorative properties of red wine and will only exacerbate your inflammations. Since there are no flavonoids to balance out the harmful effects of the alcohol, drinking beer and spirits will be detrimental to your anti-inflammatory diet and must be avoided at all costs.

Salmon

When the discussion for meat was going on, you may have wondered where fish had disappeared in that mix. Fish is not exactly white meat, it is actually the best kind of meat that you can have while you are on your anti-inflammatory diet.

There is a simple reason why fish is particularly important to your anti-inflammatory diet: omega 3 fatty acids. You have read several times over the course of this list that omega 3s are some of the most important nutrients that you can possibly eat as far as combating chronic inflammatory diseases goes.

The best fish that you can eat is perhaps salmon because it has the highest concentration of omega 3s as well as being high in protein, but other fish such as anchovies and sardines will do as well.

Salmon and these other fish can become important parts of your diet overall as they can become your primary sources of protein. Many people consider fish to be a delicacy and prefer it to other kinds of meat. You can rejoice as you will be able to incorporate a large amount of fish into your cuisine. Try to incorporate fish into your cruciferous stir fries in order to make a meal that is delicious and has all of the necessary nutrients as well.

Shiitake mushrooms

You might have heard of shiitake mushrooms because of the magical nutritional powers that they are supposed to possess. While the mushrooms themselves are not exactly magical, they do possess a huge amount of nutrients that can greatly help you to improve the overall functioning of your body.

Shiitake mushrooms have widely been considered to be the best foods to boost your immune system. As it turns out, they have robust anti-inflammatory properties as well, which means that they absolutely must be incorporated into your anti-inflammatory diet.

The great thing about shiitake mushrooms is that they do not have to be treated any differently than regular mushrooms. They cook in the exact same way, so you can just replace regular mushrooms with shiitake mushrooms and enjoy their unique taste. The similarities between shiitake mushrooms and regular mushrooms do not, however, mean that shiitake mushrooms possess the same limitations.

On the contrary, shiitake mushrooms can be used in a far more diverse manner than regular mushrooms. The best use of your shiitake mushrooms would be to add them to your fish and cruciferous vegetable stir fry to add a unique flavor to the mix.

Shrimp

You may be realizing by now that red meat is really the only kind of meat that is strongly discouraged while you are on your anti-inflammatory diet. White meat is somewhat discouraged, but it is allowed for the sake of variety. Once you have followed this diet long enough, you will actually be grateful for all of the different types of meat that it has introduced you to.

Shrimp is a great source of protein, not to mention the fact that the little crustacean is a veritable delicacy. Perhaps the single greatest thing about shrimp is that it contains a nutrient called astaxanthin. This nutrient is what gives shrimp its extraordinary anti-inflammatory properties.

Shrimp is preferable, but you can also give oysters and scallops a shot, although these kinds of shellfish tend to fall on the neutral side of things rather than the positive. Additionally, you can use shrimp to boost your protein intake or for its anti-inflammatory properties but don't go overboard with it. It contains a large amount of cholesterol, which is certainly going to do you no good. Remember, this diet is mostly vegetable and fruit based.

Spinach

There are a few vegetables, all of which are on this list that you absolutely must have in your diet. Spinach is one of them. It is perhaps second only fennel as the most nutrient dense food in this list. This density in nutrients happens to include an enormous amount of phytonutrients, fiber and protein. This means that it can provide you with practically everything that you need while you are on your anti-inflammatory diet.

Spinach is also one of the few things on this list that you can have every single day, simply because it is so easy to incorporate into your diet. You can use it as the base of practically every single salad that you can make, and you can add it to your stir fries in order to boost the nutritional value of your meals as well.

However, try not to add spinach to every single meal every single day. It may seem appealing, especially considering how healthy spinach is, but in the end it won't be worth it because the diet will end up becoming monotonous. Keep things exciting for yourself and you will be able to follow this diet indefinitely.

Sweet Potatoes

Regular potatoes are not on this list at all because if you really want to combat the chronic inflammation that is going on in your body you are going to want to avoid regular potatoes like the plague. Instead you are going to have to settle for sweet potatoes that, as it turns out, are a lot tastier at least in my opinion.

Sweet potatoes possess a lot of strong anti-inflammatory properties that stem from the deep concentration of phytonutrients that these root vegetables possess. However, stay away from sweet potato fries. The deep frying process removes the phytonutrients from the food and just makes it more food that would end up inflaming your body to a greater degree.

However, there are a lot of other ways to eat sweet potatoes so don't worry. You can have boiled sweet potatoes and baked sweet potatoes are a great choice. A lot of restaurants even offer sweet potatoes as an alternative to regular baked potatoes, which is an option you should definitely go for. Additionally, sweet potatoes can be boiled and mashed much in the same way regular potatoes can, so you can easily tackle your craving for mashed potatoes by using sweet potatoes instead.

Swiss Chard

Swiss chard is a leafy green, similar spinach and kale but different in the way it tastes. It does not possess any unique anti-inflammatory properties. Its phytonutrient composition is practically identical to that of kale and spinach and it does not provide any unique nutrients like many other foods in this list.

However, Swiss chard tastes different, and therein lies its importance in this list. You will need variety if you are going to last on this diet for more than a week. This is part of the reason why this list is so long.

When you are tired of kale and spinach, you can turn to Swiss chard instead. It's slightly more savory flavor and chewy texture can give you something new to think about while you are on your diet. The great thing about Swiss chard is that it is so versatile. It can be added to practically any salad and can even be added to smoothies if you are adventurous. Many people report that the chard ended up becoming their favorite leafy green because it offered its own unique flavor rather than spinach and kale which tend to seem bland in comparison.

Tomatoes

Once you have tomatoes in your diet, you are good to go because so much can be accomplished by adding this particular fruit to your list of foods that you can eat. Although tomato is a fruit, you are probably going to use it as more of a vegetable instead, by adding it to your salads for example.

The most important aspect of tomato that makes it such a useful part of your anti-inflammatory diet is the fact that it contains lycopene. Lycopene is particularly helpful if the particular type of chronic inflammation that you are suffering is heartburn. Lycopene, and by extension the tomato, can also help you to heal or treat a variety of cardiovascular problems as well. This boosts your overall health, making it easier for your body to tackle the inflammation that is so prevalent within it.

Tomatoes can be eaten any way you like them. You can have them raw as part of a salad, cooked as part of a curry or fried as part of a big English breakfast (minus the sausages and bacon of course!). You can even have tomato juice, which is an excellent way of getting a concentrated dose of the nutrients that tomatoes contain!

Turkey

This is another meat on this list that can be good for you while you are on your anti-inflammatory diet. However, turkey, just like chicken on this list, is not particularly effective at helping to tackle inflammation. It has only been included so that you have an alternative to beef and can get your daily requirement of protein from meat instead of from a vegetable or some kind of legume or lentil.

Most of us are addicted to meat, and without a large supply of it we would not be able to follow this diet. Turkey is a lesser evil than beef, as it satisfies your meat craving while keeping the inflammatory substances to a minimum. Just remember that if you want to eat turkey, you will absolutely have to eat the lean cuts otherwise the fat would disrupt your body's process of combating inflammation.

Additionally, it is important that you go for organic turkey wherever it is possible. This can be done most easily by avoiding turkey deli meat, because this meat is mostly full of preservatives and is not worth your time if you want to stick to your diet.

Turmeric

Once again we come back to the golden rule that if it is part of the Indian diet it is probably the best thing that you could possibly eat while you are on your anti-inflammatory diet. Turmeric is another addition to this list that is part of the Indian diet, and is by no coincidence one of the most important spices that you can add to your food while you are on your anti-inflammatory diet.

It is important to remember that while you are on your anti-inflammatory diet everything that you consume must conform to this diet. This is the only way that you would be able to facilitate an internal body chemistry that would not be conducive to inflammation. Hence, the spices that you consume must also conform to the rules of your diet. Hence, turmeric is an excellent way for you to add some flavor to your diet whilst simultaneously maintaining the internal body chemistry that you have been trying so hard to create through your anti-inflammatory diet.

In order to incorporate it into your diet, simply sprinkle it on your foods as they cook to add a bit of flavor. Most Indian curries have a lot of turmeric in them, so it is recommended that you follow Indian recipes while you are on this diet.

Turnips

You will have heard only once before in this entire list the name of the vitamin that I am about to tell you turnips contain. This vitamin is vitamin K. The fact that vitamin K is so rarely found in natural fruits and vegetables make the turnip an incredibly important part of your anti-inflammatory diet.

Turnips are also incredibly important because they contain omega 3s which, as you already know, are some of the most important nutrients that you can consume as far as your anti-inflammatory diet is concerned. The presence of both vitamin K as well as omega 3s in this vegetable are compounded by the fact that it is densely packed with vitamin C as well, rounding it off as a very useful vegetable to add to your diet.

You can cook turnip in a variety of ways, however make sure that you cook them with precision as it is easy to overdo or underdo it. You can also include turnips raw as part of your salads or blend them into smoothies.

Zucchini

Rounding of this list is the zucchini, a cousin of sorts to the cucumber. Zucchini is not as powerful as an anti-inflammatory agent when compared to the likes of spinach or kale but that does not mean that it is not an important addition to your diet.

Zucchini has strong anti-inflammatory properties as well, and is recommended as a part of your diet simply because it is one of the most popular vegetables in the world. It is important to have a varied diet so that you will not get bored after all.

Zucchini is also in this list because it is tasty. You will need all the foods you can find that are both tasty and possess anti-inflammatory properties, so if you are looking for some variety in your diet look no further than zucchini!

Zucchini is easy to serve and goes well with salads. Additionally, you can use zucchini in your cooked dishes as well. It tastes great boiled or steamed and can add a nice flavor to soup as well. Just mix things up and see how they go and before you know you will be making your very own zucchini recipes!

Conclusion To This List

This is list is all you need to go on this diet. Follow this comprehensive list of foods with precision. This list has been compiled with great care, so there should be no need to stray from it as long as you are following your anti-inflammatory diet. You will find that this list contains enough foods that you will be able to add quite a bit of variety to your diet. This can help you turn your diet into more than just a temporary thing. You can turn it into a lifestyle!

Chapter 7
Ingredients To Avoid

What follows is another list that consists of things that you should avoid while you are on this diet. The entries in this list are not foods but rather components of food. You should avoid these ingredients in food wherever possible. This list also contains foods that you should avoid.

Sugar

Sugar is at the very top of this list for a very good reason: it is one of the worst things that you can eat while you are on your anti-inflammatory diet. Our body simply was not built to digest so much sugar, and forcing so much sugar into it is, for a lack of a better word, killing it.

Hence, if you want to reduce the amount of inflammation in your body, cut down on the sweets and increase the amount of fruits you eat instead. Try to make these fruits one of the anti-inflammation foods that were mentioned in the previous list!

Cooking Oils

In the previous chapter it was recommended that you start using Extra Virgin Olive Oil as your main cooking oil. Notice how there was absolutely no other option given as far as cooking oils were concerned. This is simply because if you are not using extra virgin olive oil, you are not going to be using oils in your foods period.

The vast majority of cooking oils, from sunflower to corn to canola based cooking oils, are made of artificial ingredients. They actually damage the lining of the walls in your arteries, and once these cells begin damaging they begin to compensate by spreading further apart. This results in inflamed blood vessels which are extremely dangerous.

Hence, if you want to reduce the inflammation in your body your only choice is to cut these cooking oils out of your diet completely and replace them with extra virgin olive oil.

Trans fats

Trans fats damage cells much in the same ways that cooking oils do. This is because they are the very ingredient that makes cooking oils so deadly. However, trans fats are present in other foods as well. Commercial baked goods, fried food and even peanut butter contain this ingredient.

If you shop organic you will find that it is generally easier to buy products that are not steeped in trans fats. However, this does not mean that you will not find trans fats at all. Often companies sneak trans fats into the mix simply because it would make the food cheaper to make.

Additionally, organic food is often more expensive to buy. Hence, the best thing that you can do is to check the label of the food that you are getting before you buy it in order to make sure that it doesn't contain any trans fats.

White Bread

The thing about white bread is that it is refined. Bread never used to be white, it is a modern innovation that was invented in order to make the bread taste better and make us more liable to buy it. This works because white bread, and white grain pasta for that matter, breaks down into sugar very quickly, thereby giving your body a sugar rush. This makes your body crave it more.

However, this sugar rush that your body gets can actually lead to inflammation, particularly in your joints and blood vessels. This is an adverse reaction to the excess sugar that is in your body. As has been stated in the sugar section of this chapter, our bodies are simply not built to withstand the consumption of so much sugar.

Burgers

Burgers are the sum of everything that is absolutely incompatible with the anti-inflammatory diet. It is full of beef, which in itself is an inflammatory food, which is usually deep fried, something that fills it with even more inflammatory trans fats, and is often served with generous helpings of cheese to boot.

When we eat these saturated fats, the bacterium that is present in our digestive system alters its functioning. Our body actually triggers an immune response because it realizes how harmful the food that we are eating is.

The immune response is the inflammation that we suffer. In essence, when we eat burgers we are causing our body to shut itself down in a most literal fashion. This is simply not worth the very brief pleasant sensation that we tend to get after we have eaten a burger.

Alcohol

As you have read in the previous list, red wine is allowed in moderation but the consumption of beer and spirits is strongly discouraged. It is now important that you understand why so that you undertake this abstinence with the seriousness that it deserves.

When we consume alcohol, we make it easier for bacteria and other microbes to enter our bodies. These microbes cause inflammation to our internal organs. This inflammation is essentially a response from our immune system. The organ essentially begins to shut down so that the rest of the body remains safe.

Additionally, when we consume alcohol your body immediately breaks it down to its base form so that it doesn't harm our internal chemical balance. This base form is sugar. Essentially, when we drink alcohol we are consuming massive amounts of sugar, and you are probably well aware of how harmful sugar is while you are on your anti-inflammatory diet.

Hence, avoid the alcohol. It is better to be safe than sorry.

Omega 6 Fatty Acids

You will have heard about omega 3 fatty acids in the list in the previous chapter. Now it is time that you learned about their dangerous cousins, the omega 6 fatty acids.

Omega 6 fatty acids actually have the exact opposite effect on our body that omega 3 fatty acids have. Where omega 3 fatty acids reduce inflammation, omega 6 fatty acids tend to induce inflammation in the first place.

This is because we are overloading on this particular type of fatty acids, whilst ignoring omega 3s completely. It is this imbalance that actually ends up causing us to become inflamed from within.

In order to avoid omega 6 fatty acids, simply cut back on seeds that are rich in omega 6 acids. This basically includes absolutely any seeds apart from chia seeds. You can cut omega 6s out completely by following the list of food provided in the previous chapter.

Milk

There is something dangerous about the milk that we consume that we never seem to take into account while we are guzzling our gallons of fresh dairy: this milk is biologically incompatible with our bodies.

Think about it. Cows produce milk for baby cows, and baby cows have a vastly different biological makeup than humans. Hence, when we consume milk we are actually consuming something that our body is not ready for at all. Naturally, this leads to inflammation.

However, it is the saturated fat content in milk that actually ends up causing the inflammation in the first place. As it turns out, nonfat milk actually helps to prevent inflammation to a certain degree, so if you must consume milk make sure that it contains absolutely no fat. Even milk that has two percent fat in it would send you body over the edge.

MSG

MSG is the shortened form of monosodium glutamate, and it is a chemical that you absolutely must avoid if you want to decrease the amount of inflammation that your body is going through. In order to understand why MSG does what it does, it is important to understand what the chemical is in the first place.

MSG is essentially a preservative that is used because it tends to enhance the taste of the product that it is put in. In fact, people have reportedly preferred products with MSG in them because it tasted better. However, it is important to understand that MSG is not a chemical that occurs naturally in food. Rather, it is a chemical that was created for the express purpose of preserving food whilst simultaneously making it taste better. Hence, it is this unnatural origin of this chemical that causes inflammation in our bodies when it is consumed.

Gluten

Gluten free diets have become increasingly popular ever since it was discovered that an over consumption of gluten could lead to celiac disease. Many people that were not even diagnosed with the disease decided that it would be a good idea to take preventative measures and adopt a gluten free diet before the disease had a chance to rear its head.

As a result, they ended up feeling much better. This is because gluten causes inflammatory changes to our bodies. These changes are somewhat minor, restricted to bloating or changes in our digestive patterns, but just because something is minor for the moment does not mean that it can't become something majorly dangerous in the long run. Hence, it is highly advised that you cut gluten out of your diet if you want to follow your anti-inflammatory diet successfully.

Processed or Inorganic Meat

It was made pretty clear in the previous chapter's list that meat is not exactly an okay part of a successful anti-inflammatory diet. However, if you absolutely must eat meat, it is imperative that you avoid meats that have been processed or are inorganic.

This because processed meats are full of chemicals that will end up causing inflammation in the long run. These preservatives and other chemicals that are added to make the meat taste better should have no part in our daily diets, let alone diets designed to combat inflammation.

Inorganic meat, or meat that was derived from feedlot cows, is also dangerous because it will be full of toxins. Livestock kept in such environments invariably transfer diseases from one another, and these diseases will greatly exacerbate the amount of inflammation that your body would end up suffering through as a result.

Aspartame

Aspartame is similar to MSG in a lot of ways. Although MSG is a preservative and aspartame is an artificial sweetener, they are both similar in the fact that they were both invented by man. They are not naturally occurring chemicals, even though they are added to the food we eat.

When the health craze began to take hold, soda companies needed to make their drinks marketable to the weight watcher consumers whilst keeping them tasting good. Hence, aspartame was created. Aspartame contains all the sweetness of sugar whilst at the same time having practically none of the calories.

However, aspartame is extremely dangerous and should not be consumed. The chemical causes your body to react negatively to the point where your brain might end up getting inflamed. This is the most severe form of inflammation and could end up causing severe neurological damage in the long run.

Chapter 8

Frequently Asked Questions

Can The Anti Inflammatory Diet Help Soothe My Sciatica?

The anti-inflammatory diet is, by nature, the sort of diet that soothes inflammation. The foods that you eat soothe inflammation, and the foods that you avoid are those that would exacerbate inflammation. Hence, if you want to know about whether the anti-inflammatory diet would be able to soothe the disease that you are suffering from, you must first ascertain whether the disease involves inflammation in any way. If it does, you can be sure that the anti-inflammation diet would help to make it better.

Sciatica is the inflammation of the sciatic nerve. That in itself should give you your answer, but it is important to go in depth as far as these questions go. The anti-inflammatory diet would completely remove foods that would exacerbate this inflammation of your sciatic nerve, foods such as beef and dairy products. Once these foods are out of your diet your body will begin to heal itself, and it will be aided by the anti-inflammation supporting foods that you will be eating like spinach and kale.

However, the anti-inflammatory diet will also boost your body's ability to heal itself. The high antioxidant count of the foods you will be eating will help your body to become stronger, and might even end up reversing the negative effects of your sciatica to some degree. Just make sure that you follow the diet with accuracy and you will be better in no time.

Can The Anti Inflammatory Diet Help To Treat Fibromyalgia?

In order to answer this question it is important to first explain to you the difference between treatment and supplementation of treatment. There is enormous confusion about this topic in the healthcare industry and it is wreaking havoc with a lot of people's health.

There are a lot of conditions that can be treated with diet. However, these conditions can never be cured, and using just a diet to keep them at bay is never a good idea. The only way to really treat these conditions is using medicine because you need an aggressive approach.

Conditions such as fibromyalgia move too fast for a diet to be able to affect them in time. If you focus simply on diet you would be leaving the rest of your body high and dry, and the effects of this neglect could result in your death.

That being said, the anti-inflammatory diet can somewhat improve the symptoms of fibromyalgia. It is an inflammation based condition after all, so following this diet should make it easier for your medicine to do its job. Through a combination of medicine and diet you should be able to keep your condition at bay without any negative consequences.

However, consult your doctor before you start on this diet. It is better to be safe than sorry with these things after all, and your specific condition might have some unknown side effects that would be exacerbated by you adopting this diet.

Can I Soothe My Toothache By Eating Anti-Inflammatory Foods?

Toothaches are caused by inflammation, and following the anti-inflammatory diet would help remove this pain. However, this is mostly due to the fact that the anti-inflammation diet cuts sugar completely out of your diet. Sugar is the main cause of toothache, so if you are suffering from one you don't have to worry about following the entire anti-inflammatory diet. Simply cut the sugar out of your diet and your toothache should subside. If it persists, go and see a dentist, as the diet will not be able to help the problem that is causing your pain.

Will Following The Anti Inflammatory Diet Help Me To Treat My Hemorrhoids?

Hemorrhoids are essentially inflammations, which mean that you can definitely treat them by applying the rules of the anti-inflammatory diet. However, it is important to understand that improvement in your hemorrhoids will certainly not be easy to attain. You will have to follow this diet for a significant period of time. If you do not experience any improvement after a period of two weeks it is highly recommended that you go and see a doctor lest the problem get out of hand.

What Are The Most Effective Anti-Inflammatory Foods?

The list provided in this book is comprehensive, but you might be looking for specifics. The absolute best foods with the strongest anti-inflammatory qualities are kale, wild salmon, garlic, onions, extra virgin olive oil and turmeric. If you really want to get the inflammation down or just can't stand the pain anymore and need quick results, go for these foods. A wild salmon stir fry in EVOO with garlic and onions with a little kale on the side can give you all of the anti-inflammatory juice you'll need!

Should I Take Anti Inflammatory Drugs?

This is a very important question. There used to be a wide variety of anti-inflammatory drugs that were available which supposedly helped a great deal as far as inflammation was concerned. However, these drugs had adverse side effects and were taken off the market fairly quickly. Hence, it is important for you to ask your doctor before you take any anti-inflammatory medication. The risk of adverse side effects is far too high for you to be able to risk taking over the counter anti-inflammatory medication, especially if you are following an anti-inflammatory diet.

Can Following The Anti Inflammatory Diet Reduce Pain And Swelling?

It is true that eating foods with anti-inflammatory properties can, in fact, reduce pain and swelling over time. However, if you need immediate relief you will need to take anti-inflammatory drugs. Just be sure to be careful lest the drugs you take end up causing unwanted side effects. Remember to keep your doctor in the loop about everything, from your swelling to your diet to the fact that you are going to start taking anti-inflammatory drugs to combat the pain and swelling.

Will I Gain Weight On The Anti Inflammatory Diet?

To put this simply, it is very difficult to gain weight while you are on the anti-inflammatory diet. This is simply because the foods that you are going to be eating won't allow it. The only way you would gain weight while you are on the diet is if you cheat, since everything down to the size of your portions is controlled in your diet. In fact, you are probably going to end up losing weight while you are on the anti-inflammatory diet.

Is The Anti Inflammatory Diet Effective

This question is important. You need proof that the diet you are following is effective, otherwise why on earth would you follow it? There is a significant body of work that supports the claim that eating these foods, and avoiding others, will cause a decrease in chronic inflammation in your body. If you are truly concerned about the efficacy of this diet, just go and ask your doctor about it. He or she will confirm that the foods listed in this book will help to reduce chronic inflammation in your body.

Will I Get Constipated On The Anti Inflammatory Diet?

The way the diet is built will actually encourage you to end up eating more fiber. This means that if you follow this diet, you actually will start having regular bowel movements rather than getting constipated. As long as you follow this diet as it is specified you should have absolutely no problems with constipation. However, if you do start getting constipated, go and see a doctor. You might be having a negative reaction to the foods that you are eating.

How Well Does The Diet Conform To Generally Accepted Dietary Guidelines?

Let us look at how the anti-inflammatory diet ticks all the necessary boxes, when it comes to the dietary guidelines.

Fat:

The diet prescribes only the consumption of 30% of total calories from fat. The government recommends that the ideal consumption of fat should contribute to only 20 to 35 percent of the total calories. The typical American diet makes you consume so much fat that it contributes to at least 55% of the total calories. To reduce the intake of diet, here are a few pointers:

•   Reduce the consumption of saturated fats. In other words, reduce the intake of cream, high fat cheese, fatty meats, butter and chicken (without skin removed).

•   Avoid foods made with palm kernel oil.

•   Avoid the usage of mixed vegetable oils, corn oil, and sunflower oil, cottonseed oil and safflower oils while cooking.

Use extra virgin olive oil for cooking instead. You can also use expeller pressed organic version of canola oil.

• Avoid the usage of vegetable shortenings, margarine in your diet. In fact, avoid any foods that are made with hydrogenated oils.

Carbohydrates:

The dietary guidelines suggest that only 45% to 65% of the calories should come from carbohydrates. This diet fails to hit the mark for only 31% of the calories are derived from carbohydrates when you follow this diet. To meet the requirement, eat more beans, sweet potatoes and winter squashes.

Proteins:

When you follow this diet, you derive up to 14% of calories from proteins. This is within the government's recommendation that 10% to 35% of calories should be derived from proteins. To increase your intake of proteins, here are a few pointers:

• Eat more vegetable protein. In other words, increase your consumption of soy foods.

• Eat generous quantities of natural cheese and yogurt.

Salt:

The typical American diet is loaded with salt. The prescribed intake of salt is a maximum of 2,300 milligrams in a day. If you are over 51 years old and have hypertension, the prescribed intake is only 1,500 milligrams a day. However, this diet makes you consume up to 3,317 milligrams a day. Hence, go light on your salt when you cook to ensure that you do not consume salt more than the prescribed levels.

Potassium:

Potassium is a very essential nutrient. It plays an important role in countering the ability of salt to increase blood pressure. It also plays a key role in reducing the risk of developing kidney stones and decreasing bone loss. The prescribed intake of potassium is at least 4,700 mg a day, which is quite high. Most diets fail to meet this mark. The anti-inflammatory diet is no exception to this. It provides for only 1,555 milligrams of this essential nutrient. Hence, include more of foods rich in potassium such as bananas.

Calcium:

Calcium is another essential nutrient. The body requires calcium not just for the purpose of building and maintaining bones but also for ensuring that the blood vessels function properly. It also plays an important role in ensuring that the muscles function properly. The prescribed intake of calcium is around 1,000 mg to 1,300 mg a day. This diet almost hits the mark by providing 833 mg of calcium a day.

Fiber:

The recommended intake of fiber is between 22 and 34 grams. This diet is packed with fiber for it prescribes the intake of fruits, vegetables, whole grains and beans in generous quantities. Hence, it provides for 40 grams of fiber.

Vitamin B 12:

Vitamin B 12 is another vital nutrient that plays a key role in facilitating proper cell metabolism. You are required to consume at least 2.4 micrograms of this nutrient to ensure that your cell metabolism is good. This diet encourages the consumption of eggs, yogurt, salmon and trout, which are naturally rich in this nutrient. This diet provides for 9.3 micrograms of this nutrient.

Vitamin D:

If you are not exposed to enough sunlight, you are expected to consume at least 15 micrograms of this nutrient. Consumption of this nutrient is important for it reduces the risk of bone fractures. However, this diet lacks in vitamin D.

How Easy Is The Diet To Follow?

This diet is not as difficult as the other diet plans available in the market. It is relatively easier for it does not impose strict guidelines. There is a lot of flexibility involved, which makes it easy for you to adapt to this diet plan without much hassles. Some of the reasons why this diet plan is easier to follow are as follows:

•   There are tons of anti-inflammatory diet recipes out there that can make this dieting a pleasant experience. Even though some of the recipes involve a lot of preparation time, the cooking time is considerably low, which makes it easier to whip out these dishes.

•   It does not prohibit you from eating out in restaurants. The only catch is that you need to check out the menu beforehand to ensure that you consume only those foods that are anti-inflammatory in nature. The Japanese cuisine is highly recommended for it is mostly anti-inflammatory in nature.

•   It also allows the consumption of alcohol. Hence, people are not expected to give up alcohol, as in the case with most of the other diets.

•   The diet makes you consume at least 2,000 calories and up to 3,000 calories a day. Moreover, it is packed with fiber. Hence, you don't feel hungry often, when you follow this diet.

- There is no lack for flavors, when it comes to this diet. In other words, it is not a boring and bland diet. It is, in fact, packed with vibrant flavors.

-

Does This Diet Have Cardiovascular Benefits?

Yes. This diet certainly does have cardiovascular benefits for it reduces the risk for several heart diseases. It is also proven that this diet reduces the bad LDL cholesterol levels in our blood. Research also shows that this diet can reduce blood pressure.

Even though, inflammation is not a reason for cardiovascular diseases, it is a common phenomenon among patients suffering from heart diseases. This is because, according to studies, there is a correlation between elevated levels of C-reactive protein and heart diseases. The C-reactive protein (CRP) is the protein present in our blood levels that triggers inflammation. This is why most people suffering from cardiovascular diseases suffer from inflammation.

The CRP levels also indicate the individual's risk of contracting cardiac diseases. Several medical trials and studies show that these CRP levels can be tackled by fiber. This diet is packed with fiber, which reduces the CRP levels in blood, thereby reducing inflammation and the risk of cardiac diseases.

Are There Any Health Risks Associated With This Diet?

No, there are no health risks associated with following this diet. However, if you are suffering from any medical condition, you should first consult with your doctor about the compatibility of this diet with your medication.

Chapter 9
Breakfast Recipes

In this chapter, I have some exciting breakfast recipes for you. Begin your day on an exciting note!

I.   Cinnamon Almond Baked Oatmeal

Ingredients:

• 4 cups of rolled oats, gluten free

• 3 teaspoons of baking powder

• Pinch of sea salt

• 4 ½ cups of almond or coconut milk

• 8 tablespoons of honey or pure maple syrup

• 2 teaspoons of vanilla extract

• 2 teaspoons of ground cinnamon

• 8 tablespoons of sunflower seeds

- 8 tablespoons of dried cranberries or blueberries

- 2 teaspoons of ground flax seeds

- 4 tablespoons of sunflower seed butter

- Coconut oil

Instructions:

1. Preheat the oven to 375 degrees F.

2. Use coconut oil to grease 12 ramekins and keep aside.

3. Take a large bowl. Add the oats, sea salt and baking powder to the bowl and mix well.

4. Take a small bowl. Add the coconut milk, maple syrup and vanilla extract to the bowl and mix well.

5. Pour the coconut milk mixture on top of the oats mixture in the large bowl and mix well. Ensure that the coconut milk mixture is evenly distributed.

6. Add the ground cinnamon to the mixture and combine well.

7. Distribute the mixture evenly among the 12 cups.

8. Garnish the cups with the sunflower seeds and dried cranberries.

9. Place the cups in the oven and bake them for around 30 minutes. This should give enough time for it to turn golden brown in color.

10. At the end of thirty minutes, remove the cups from the oven. Sprinkle the flax seeds on top of the cups.

11. Drizzle sunflower seed butter on top of the muffins. Return the cups to the oven. Let it cook in the oven for an additional two minutes.

12. At the end of two minutes, remove the cups from the oven. Keep the cups aside for at least twenty minutes. This should be enough time for the muffins to cool.

13. Serve them warm.

II.   Cherry Coconut Porridge

Ingredients:

- 8 tablespoons of chia seeds

- 3 cups of oats

- 6 tablespoons of raw cacao

- 6 to 8 cups of coconut milk

- Coconut shavings

- Fresh cherries

- 2 tablespoons of maple syrup

- Dark chocolate shavings

- Pinch of stevia

Instructions:

1.   Take a medium sized saucepan. Add the coconut milk, chia seeds, oats, stevia and cacao to it. Over medium heat, bring the mixture to a boil. Once it starts boiling, lower the heat. Allow the mixture to simmer till the oats are cooked well.

2.   Transfer the cooked oats mixture to a large bowl.

3.   Add the coconut shavings and cherries to the bowl and mix well.

4.   Pour the maple syrup on top of the contents of the bowl.

Garnish with the dark chocolate shavings and serve immediately.

5.

III.   Chia Lemon Quinoa Bowl

Ingredients:

- 2 cups of quinoa

- 3 cups of almond milk

- 9 tablespoons of pure maple syrup or honey

- 6 tablespoons of almonds, slivered thinly

- 2 tablespoons of chia seeds

- ½ teaspoon of sea salt

- Pinch of fresh lemon zest

- 4 cups of water

Instructions:

1.   Take a medium sized pot. Add the water to it. Now, add in the quinoa and bring the water to a boil, over medium high heat.

2.   As the water begins to boil, reduce the heat to low. Cover the lid of the pot and allow the quinoa to simmer in the pot for

at least 15 to 20 minutes. This should be enough time for the quinoa to get cooked well.

3.   At the end of twenty minutes, remove the pot from the heat. Keep the lid covered and allow the quinoa to rest for another five minutes.

4.   Remove the lid. Use a fork to fluff the quinoa and transfer it to a large bowl.

5.   Add the chia seeds, slivered almonds, sea salt and lemon zest to bowl and mix well.

6.   Pour the almond milk and maple syrup into the bowl next and mix well.

7.   Serve warm.

IV.   Creamy Millet Porridge

Ingredients:

- 2 cups of uncooked millet

- 2 cups of almond milk

- 1 cup of raw almonds

- 2 teaspoons of maple syrup

- 2 teaspoons of butter, dairy free and vegan

- 2 tablespoons of carob powder

- 4 tablespoons of cinnamon

- 4 tablespoons of coconut flakes

- 4 tablespoons of ground flax seeds

- ½ teaspoon of almond extract

- ½ teaspoon of sea salt

- Water

Instructions:

1.   Preheat the oven to 375 degrees F.

2.   Place the millet in a colander. Use cool water to rinse the millet. This will ensure that dirt and debris from the millet are removed.

3.   Take a medium sized pot. Add water to the pot. Transfer the millet to the pot.

4.   Keep stirring the millet and bring the water to a boil.

5.   Once the water starts boiling, reduce the heat to low. Allow the millet to simmer in the pot for at least 20 minutes. This should be enough time for the millet to absorb the water.

6.   At the end of 20 minutes, remove the pot from the heat. Keep the lid covered and let the millet cook inside the pot for another five minutes.

7.   At the end of five minutes, use a fork to fluff the millet and keep aside.

8.   Take a large bowl. Add the almonds, maple syrup, carob powder and butter to the bowl and mix well. Ensure that the almonds are coated evenly.

9.   Line a baking sheet with parchment paper. Spread the almond mixture evenly on the baking sheet.

10.   Place the baking sheet in the oven and bake it for 30 minutes. This should be enough time for the almonds to get roasted.

11.   As the almonds are getting roasted, transfer the cooked millet to eight serving bowls.

12.   Add the almond milk, flax seeds, toasted almonds, almond extract, sea salt and coconut flakes to the serving bowls and mix well. Serve warm.

V. Mushroom And Baby Spinach Frittata

Ingredients:

- 2 medium onions, finely diced

- 2 teaspoons of fresh rosemary

- 2 teaspoons of garlic, minced finely

- 1 pound fresh mushrooms, finely chopped

- 2 tablespoons of water

- 20 ounces of fresh baby spinach

- 5 cups of egg substitute

- ½ cup of goat cheese, crumbled

- 1 teaspoon of fresh black pepper

- Vegetable cooking spray

Instructions:

1. Preheat the oven to 350 degrees F.

2. Wash the baby spinach well to ensure that it is free of dirt. Cut it into small pieces.

3.   Using cooking spray, grease a medium sized skillet. Place the skillet over medium high heat.

4.   Add the diced onions and garlic to the skillet and sauté it for around five minutes. This should be enough time for the onions to become tender.

5.   Add the rosemary and chopped mushrooms to the skillet and mix well. Cook the mixture for another five minutes.

6.   Now, add the chopped spinach to the skillet and keep cooking for another 3 minutes. This should be sufficient time for the spinach leaves to wilt.

7.   Remove the skillet from the heat and allow the mushroom mixture to cool.

8.   Take a large bowl. Add the egg substitute and pepper to the bowl and mix well. Now, add in the mushroom and spinach mixture to the bowl and mix well.

9.   Add the goat cheese to the bowl and mix well.

10.   Clean the skillet well and grease it with cooking spray. Return the skillet to the stove and turn on the heat to medium high.

11.   Add the egg mixture to the skillet and keep stirring it for one minute.

12.   Bake the egg mixture for around 15 to 20 minutes. This should be sufficient time of the mixture to set.

13.   Remove the frittata from the oven and allow it to cool for five minutes. Cut into wedges and serve warm.

VI.   Apple Muesli With Goji Berries

Ingredients:

- 2 cups of rolled oats

- 4 large apples

- 6 tablespoons of flax seeds

- 1 cup of dried Goji berries

- 2 ½ cups of coconut water

- 4 tablespoons of fresh mint leaves, chopped coarsely

- 2 ½ cups of Greek yogurt

- 6 tablespoons of honey

- Pinch of salt

- Chopped nuts, for garnish

- Chopped berries, for garnish

- Granola, for garnish

Instructions:

1. Take a large bowl. Grate the apples over the bowl. Stop grating once you have reached the core.

2. Add the rolled oats, flax seeds, mint and goji berries to the bowl and mix well.

3. Pour the coconut water and yogurt into the bowl and mix well. Keep stirring till the ingredients mix well.

4. Cover the bowl and place it in the refrigerator. Allow the muesli to rest in the refrigerator overnight.

5. Take a small bowl. Add the honey and salt to the bowl and mix well.

6. Add the honey mixture to the muesli and mix well.

7. Transfer the muesli to serving bowls. Garnish the muesli with the chopped berries, nuts and granola and serve immediately.

VII. Vanilla Millet Muffin

Ingredients:

- 2 eggs

- 2 teaspoons of baking powder

- 1 teaspoon of vanilla extract

- 3 cups of millet

- ½ cup of coconut oil, melted

- 2/3 cups of sugar

Instructions:

1. Preheat the oven to 350 degrees F.

2. Grease two muffin tins and keep aside.

3. Place the millet in a colander. Use cool water to rinse the millet. This will ensure that dirt and debris from the millet are removed.

4. Take a medium sized pot. Add water to the pot. Transfer the millet to the pot.

5. Keep stirring the millet and bring the water to a boil.

6.   Once the water starts boiling, reduce the heat to low. Allow the millet to simmer in the pot for at least 20 minutes. This should be enough time for the millet to absorb the water.

7.   At the end of 20 minutes, remove the pot from the heat. Keep the lid covered and let the millet cook inside the pot for another five minutes.

8.   At the end of five minutes, use a fork to fluff the millet and keep aside.

9.   Take a large bowl. Add the vanilla extract, egg and coconut oil to the bowl and mix well.

10.   Add the cooked millet, sugar and baking powder to the bowl of a blender. Blend it on medium speed.

11.   As the millet mixture is getting blended in the blender, add in the egg mixture slowly. Keep blending till you get a smooth batter.

12.   Divide the batter among the cups in the muffin tins.

13.   Place the tins in the oven and bake for around 30 minutes. This should be enough time for the muffins to turn light brown in color.

14.   At the end of thirty minutes, place the muffin tins in the rack and allow it to cool.

15. Serve the muffins warm!

VIII. Coconut Milk Rice Pudding With Ginger And Citrus

Ingredients:

- 2 cups of water

- 2 cans of coconut milk

- 1 ½ cups of orange juice

- ¼ teaspoon of salt

- 4 teaspoons of vanilla extract

- 4 to 8 tablespoons of maple syrup, to taste

- 2 teaspoons of ground ginger

- 2 cups of long grain basmati rice

- 2 tablespoons of orange zest

- 2 teaspoons of cinnamon

Instructions:

1.   Take a large pot. Add the water, coconut milk, vanilla extract, rice, orange juice and salt to the pot.

2.   Bring the mixture to a boil. Once it starts boiling, reduce the heat and allow the mixture to simmer, with the lid covered. Ensure that the lid does not completely cover the pot, to let some steam out.

3.   Allow the mixture to simmer for around 30 minutes or until the rice has absorbed all the liquid.

4.   At the end of 30 minutes, stir in the ginger, maple syrup, orange zest and cinnamon.

5.   Continue cooking the rice mixture in the pot until it turns soft and creamy. Add more syrup or water, if you don't get the desired consistency.

6.   Remove the pot from the heat and transfer the pudding to serving bowls. Serve warm.

Chapter 10
Main Course Recipes

Now that you have learnt the key to beginning your day on a healthy note, let's get on with some main course recipes that will help you stay on the track throughout the day.

I.   White Bean And Chicken Chili Blanca

Ingredients:

- 4 tablespoons of extra-virgin olive oil

- 2 pounds of skinless chicken breasts

- 2 medium onions, finely diced

- 4 garlic cloves

- 4 15-ounce cans white beans, rinsed and drained

- 2 cups of fresh corn kernels

- 2 4-ounce cans of green chilies, chopped

- 4 teaspoons of ground cumin

- 4 teaspoons of pure chili powder

- ¼ teaspoon of cayenne pepper

- 6 cups of water

- 4 cups of Monterey Jack cheese, finely grated

- 4 tablespoons of fresh cilantro, finely chopped

- Salt

- Pepper

Instructions:

1. Season the chicken breasts well with pepper and salt. Set aside.

2. Take a large saucepan. Pour the oil into it and turn the heat to high. Once the pan is hot, add the seasoned chicken breasts to the pan and let it cook for around three minutes. This should be enough time for the chicken breasts to cook nicely.

3. Once the breasts are browned, reduce the heat to medium. Add the chopped onions and garlic to the pan. Cook for around five to six minutes or till the onions turn translucent.

4. Add the chopped chilies, cumin, chili powder, cayenne pepper, beans, water and corn to the pan. Bring the mixture to a boil. Once the mixture starts boiling, reduce the heat to low. Allow the mixture to simmer, uncovered, for at least one hour.

5. At the end of one hour, remove the pan from the heat. Transfer the mixture to serving bowls.

6. Garnish each serving with the chopped cilantro and grated cheese. Serve warm.

II. Roasted Chicken With Balsamic Vinaigrette

Ingredients:

- ½ cup of balsamic vinegar

- 4 tablespoons of Dijon mustard

- 4 tablespoons of fresh lemon juice

- 4 garlic cloves, finely chopped

- 4 tablespoons of olive oil

- Salt

- Freshly ground black pepper

- 2 whole chickens

- 2 teaspoons of lemon zest

- 2 tablespoons of fresh parsley leaves, finely chopped

Instructions:

1. Cut the chicken into smaller pieces. Keep aside the neck, backbone and giblets.

2. Take a small bowl. Add the mustard, garlic, vinegar, olive oil, lemon juice, pepper and salt to the bowl. Mix well.

3. Place the chicken pieces in a large airtight bag. Add the vinaigrette to the bag as well and let it mix with the chicken pieces. Seal the bag and place it in the refrigerator. Allow it to rest there for at least 2 hours.

4. Preheat the oven to 400 degrees F.

5. Grease a baking dish. Remove the marinated chicken from the refrigerator and arrange it on the baking dish.

6. Place the dish in the oven and cook the chicken for an hour. If you notice that the chicken is getting browned too quickly, wrap it in foil and cook it. This should be sufficient time for the chicken to get roasted.

7. At the end of one hour, transfer the roasted chicken to a platter.

8. Garnish the chicken pieces with the lemon zest and chopped parsley and serve hot.

III. Arctic Char With Sweet Potato Puree And Chinese Broccoli

Ingredients:

- 6 red skinned sweet potatoes

- 2 teaspoons of hot Chinese mustard

- 2 cups of balsamic vinegar

- 3 teaspoons of soy sauce

- 2 pounds of Chinese broccoli

- 4 slices of bacon

- 4 teaspoons of yellow mustard seeds

- 8 6 ounce arctic char fillets

- 4 tablespoons of vegetable oil

- Water

- Salt

- Freshly ground black pepper

Instructions:

1.   Preheat the oven to 400 degrees F.

2.   Wrap the sweet potatoes neatly using a foil paper. Place them in the oven and roast for at least 1 ½ hours. This should be sufficient time for the sweet potatoes to turn tender.

3.   As the sweet potatoes are roasting in the oven, wash the broccoli well. Remove the outer leaves and cut it crosswise into smaller slices. Keep aside.

4.   Ensure that the bacon slices are cut into one inch cubes.

5.   Take a large pot. Add some water and salt to it. Once the water starts boiling, add the broccoli slices to the pot and cook for a minute. This should be sufficient time for the broccoli to turn tender. Remove the pot from the heat and drain the water. Keep the cooked broccoli aside.

6.   Take a medium sized skillet. Add the bacon slices to it and cook over a medium heat. Keep cooking till the edges are crisp. Transfer the cooked bacon pieces to paper towels to drain.

7.   Once the sweet potatoes have turned tender, remove them from the oven. Let it cool for a few minutes before you start peeling their skins off. Cut the sweet potatoes in halves and add the pieces to a food processor. Keep blending till it turns into a fine puree.

8.   Add six cups of the puree to a microwave friendly bowl. Add the mustard to the bowl and stir well. Season the puree well with salt. Allow the mixture to rest.

9.   Take a small saucepan. Add the vinegar to the pan and bring it to a boil. Boil it for around eight minutes till it reduces to one cup. Add the soy sauce to the pan and stir well. Remove the pan from the heat once the vinegar and soy sauce have mixed well.

10.   Add the mustard seeds to a spice grinder and process it till it is ground coarsely.

11.   Season the fish fillets well with salt and pepper.

12.   Now, garnish the fillets with the ground mustard seeds. Set aside.

13.   As the fillets are resting, take a large skillet. Add two tablespoons of oil to it and heat it over medium high heat.

14.   Add the fish fillets to the skillet and cook each side for around three minutes. Ensure that the mustard side is down when you place the fillet in the pan. Remove the fillets from the pan once the fillets turn brown and are opaque in the center.

15.   As the fillets are getting cooked, warm the sweet potato puree in the oven.

16.   Take another large skillet. Add two tablespoons of oil to it and heat it. Add the cooked broccoli and bacon pieces to it and sauté it till they are heated throughout. Remove them from the heat and season well with salt and pepper.

17.   Divide the fillets, sweet potato puree and broccoli mixture among eight plates. Drizzle with the balsamic reduction and serve warm.

IV.   Pan Seared Salmon On Baby Arugula

Ingredients:

- 4 6 ounce center-cut salmon fillets

- 3 tablespoons of fresh lemon juice

- 3 tablespoons of olive oil

- Salt, to taste

- Freshly ground black pepper, to taste

For the salad:

- 6 cups of baby arugula leaves

- 1 1/3 cups of cherry tomatoes, cut in halves

- ½ cup of red onions, thinly slivered

- Salt, to taste

- Freshly ground black pepper, to taste

- 2 tablespoons of extra-virgin olive oil

- 2 tablespoons of red wine vinegar

Instructions:

1. Take a shallow bowl. Arrange the salmon fillets neatly in it.

2. Add the lemon juice, salt, olive oil and pepper to the bowl and toss well. Ensure that the fillets are coated evenly with the lemon juice mixture. Allow the fillets to rest for at least fifteen minutes.

3. Take a large skillet. Place the fillets in the skillet and cook it for around two to three minutes, over medium high heat. Ensure that the skin side is down when you place the fillets in the pan.

4. At the end of 3 minutes, reduce the heat to medium. Cover the pan with a lid and cook the salmon fillets for another three to four minutes. This will ensure that the fillets are cooked throughout. You will notice that the skin has become crisp while the flesh has been cooked to medium rare. Remove the fillets from the heat.

5. As the cooked fillets are resting, take a small bowl. Add the tomatoes, arugula and onions to it and combine well.

6. Add the vinegar, oil, salt and pepper to it and toss well.

7. Serve the fillets warm with the salad on the side.

V.   Indian Spiced Carrot Soup

Ingredients:

- 2 teaspoons of coriander seeds

- 1 teaspoon of yellow mustard seeds

- 6 tablespoons of peanut oil

- 1 teaspoon of curry powder

- 2 tablespoons of fresh ginger, peeled and finely minced

- 4 cups of finely chopped onions

- 3 pounds of carrots

- 3 teaspoons of finely grated lime peel

- 10 cup of low-salt vegetable broth or chicken broth

- 4 teaspoons of fresh lime juice

- Plain yogurt, for garnish

- Salt, to taste

- Freshly ground black pepper, to taste

Instructions:

1. Wash the carrots well. Peel their skins off. Cut them into thin rounds and keep aside.

2. Add the mustard seeds and coriander seeds to a spice mill. Grind it till they turn into a fine powder.

3. Take a large and heavy pot. Add the oil to it and heat it over medium high heat.

4. First, add the ground mustard and coriander seeds to the pot followed by the curry powder. Stir continuously for one minute.

5. Add the minced ginger and chopped onions to the pot next.

6. Now, add the carrot slices to the pot.

7. Sprinkle salt and pepper on top of the contents of the pot.

8. Keep cooking the mixture in the pot till the onions turn translucent. This should be done in around three to four minutes.

9. Once the onions have softened, add the chicken or vegetable broth to the pot and heat it. Once the mixture starts boiling, reduce the heat to medium low.

10. Allow the mixture to simmer for around thirty minutes. This should be sufficient time for the carrots to get cooked and turn tender.

11. At the end of 30 minutes, remove the pot from the heat. Allow the soup to cool for a few minutes.

12. Transfer some of the soup to a blender and puree it nicely. Repeat this step till the entire soup is pureed.

13. Return the pureed soup to the pot. Add the lime juice to it and mix well. If the mixture is too thick, you may add in some more broth. Keep mixing till the soup reaches the desired consistency.

14. Season the soup well with salt and pepper.

15. Divide the soup among serving bowls. Garnish each bowl with the yogurt and serve hot.

VI. Tropical Quinoa Salad With Cashew Nuts

Ingredients:

- 2 cups of dried quinoa

- 1 red onion, chopped finely

- 2 cups of apple, deseeded and finely chopped

- Juice from 2 limes

- 4 tablespoons of agave or honey

- 2 tablespoons of extra-virgin olive oil

- 2 large mangoes, chopped into smaller pieces

- ½ cup of fresh mint, chopped finely

- 2 teaspoons of sea salt, to taste

- freshly ground black pepper, to taste

- 1 inch piece of ginger, chopped finely

- 2 avocadoes

- 2 cups of cashews, chopped coarsely

- 6 cups of Romaine lettuce

- 4 cups of water

- ½ cup of fresh cilantro, finely chopped

Instructions:

1. Let us prepare the vegetables before we begin cooking. Wash the lettuce well to ensure that there is no dirt. Chop the lettuce coarsely.

2. Wash the avocadoes well. Peel their skins off and cut them in halves. Remove the pits and chop them into smaller pieces.

3. Before you begin cooking the quinoa, ensure that it is rinsed well.

4. Take a medium sized pot. Add the water to it. Now, add in the quinoa and bring the water to a boil, over medium high heat.

5. As the water begins to boil, reduce the heat to low. Cover the lid of the pot and allow the quinoa to simmer in the pot for at least 15 to 20 minutes. This should be enough time for the quinoa to get cooked well.

6. At the end of twenty minutes, remove the pot from the heat. Keep the lid covered and allow the quinoa to rest for another five minutes.

7. Remove the lid. Use a fork to fluff the quinoa and transfer it to a large bowl. Let it cool for at least ten minutes.

8. Once the quinoa is cooled, add the chopped onions and carrot to the large bowl and mix well.

9. Take a small bowl. Add the olive oil, honey and lime juice to the bowl and whisk well.

10. Add the dressing to the contents of the large bowl and mix well.

11. Add the chopped mangoes to the bowl next and mix well.

12. Add the chopped cilantro, mint, ginger, pepper and salt to the bowl next and mix well.

13. Divide the salad among 8 serving bowls. Garnish each bowl with avocado pieces and cashew nuts.

14. Add the chopped lettuce to the bowl before serving. Serve at room temperature.

VII. Lentil Vegetable Soup

Ingredients:

- 2 pounds of dry French green lentils

- 6 large onions, peeled and chopped

- 8 cups of finely chopped leeks

- 6 cloves of garlic, finely minced

- ½ cup of olive oil

- 2 tablespoons of kosher salt

- 3 teaspoons of freshly ground black pepper

- 2 tablespoons of finely minced fresh thyme leaves

- 2 teaspoons of ground cumin

- 16 stalks of celery

- 8 to 12 carrots

- 6 quarts of chicken stock

- ½ cup of tomato paste

- 4 tablespoons of red wine vinegar

- Freshly grated Parmesan cheese

- Water

Instructions:

1. Wash the celery stalks well. Dice the stalks finely and keep aside.

2. Wash the carrots well and peel their skins off. Dice them into smaller pieces.

3. Take a large bowl. Add the lentils to the bowl. Pour some boiling water on top of the lentils. Allow the lentils to sit in the bowl for at least fifteen minutes. Drain the water at the end of fifteen minutes. Set aside.

4. Take a large stockpot. Add the olive oil to it and heat it over medium heat. Add the chopped onions, garlic and leeks to it. Add the cumin, thyme, pepper and salt to the pot and sauté for around 20 minutes. This should be sufficient time for the vegetables to get cooked well and turn tender.

5. Add the diced celery and carrots to the pot and sauté it for another ten minutes.

6. Now, pour the chicken stock and tomato paste into the pot and mix well.

7.   Next, add the lentils to the pot. Cover the lid of the pot and bring its contents to a boil. Remove the lid once it starts boiling and allow the mixture to simmer for around one hour. This should be sufficient time for the lentils to get cooked well.

8.   Add the red wine to the pot and mix well. Garnish the soup with grated parmesan cheese and serve hot.

VIII. Dressed Salmon

Ingredients:

- 8 skinless salmon fillets

- 1 seedless cucumber

- 4 small plum tomatoes

- 2 shallots

- 4 tablespoons of Dijon mustard

- 4 tablespoons of sugar

- ½ cup of white wine vinegar

- 1 cup of extra-virgin olive oil, plus some for drizzling

- ½ cup of fresh dill, chopped finely

- Salt

- Freshly ground black pepper

- Seafood seasoning

Instructions:

1. Wash the cucumber well and peel its skin off. Dice the cucumber finely into smaller pieces.

2. Wash the tomatoes well and cut them in halves. Remove the seeds and chop them into smaller pieces.

3. Peel the shallots and chop them into smaller pieces.

4. Take a large bowl. Add the chopped tomatoes, cucumber to the bowl and mix well.

5. Add half the shallots to the bowl and combine well. Set aside.

6. Take a small bowl. Add the white wine vinegar, mustard, sugar and the remaining shallots to the bowl. Whisk well. Add in the olive oil as you continue whisking.

7. Add the chopped dill to the bowl and mix well. Season the dressing well with salt and pepper.

8. Now take the fillets. Season it well with the seafood seasoning and black pepper. Set aside.

9.   Take a non stick skillet. Drizzle with the olive oil and heat the skillet over medium high heat. Place the seasoned fillets on the skillet and cook it for three to four minutes. This should be sufficient time for the fillets to turn golden and crispy at the edges. Now, flip the sides and cook the other side for another four minutes. This should be sufficient time for the center to turn opaque.

10.   Transfer the cooked fillets to the serving plates. Top the fillets with the tomato cucumber relish. Garnish with the dill dressing and serve warm.

Chapter 11

Dessert Recipes

Here is an opportunity to end your day on a healthy and sweet note. I have highlighted eight exciting dessert recipes.

I.   Buche De Noel

Ingredients:

For the sponge cake:

- 6 tablespoons of whole and unrefined cane sugar, divided

- Pinch of unrefined sea salt

- zest of 1 orange

- 6 pastured eggs, separated

- ¼ teaspoon of cream of tartar

- 1 teaspoon of vanilla extract

- Coconut oil or butter

- ½ cup of cocoa powder

For the filling:

- 1 teaspoon of unrefined cane sugar

- 1 vanilla bean

- 1 ½ cups of raw heavy cream

Instructions:

1. Preheat the oven to 375 degrees F.

2. Cut parchment paper in such a fashion that it fits inside the jelly roll pan.

3. Use the coconut oil or butter to grease the parchment paper. Now, proceed to dust the paper with the cocoa powder.

4. Line the jelly roll pan with the parchment paper.

5. Take a large bowl. Add the egg yolks, sea salt, cocoa powder, four tablespoons of unrefined cane sugar, orange zest and vanilla extract to the bowl and whisk well. Keep whisking till the mixture turns thickened, smooth and creamy.

6. Take another bowl. Add the egg whites, cream of tartar and the remaining unrefined cane sugar and beat well. Keep beating till you get soft peaks.

7. Now, fold the eggs white mixture into the yolk and cocoa mixture. Ensure that the mixtures combine well.

8. Pour the prepared batter over the parchment lined in the jelly roll pan.

9. Place the pan in the oven and bake the batter for at least 15 minutes. At the end of 15 minutes, remove the pan from the oven and let the cake to cool.

10. While the cake is cooling, let's get started with the filling. Take another bowl. Add the heavy cream, unrefined cane sugar and contents of the vanilla bean to it and whisk well. Keep whisking well till soft peaks form. Keep it aside.

11. Now, dust the cake with cocoa powder.

12. Once the cake has cooled enough, invert it over a kitchen towel slowly.

13. Proceed to spread the whipped cream on the cake. Place the cake on a serving platter, with its seam down.

14. Gently slice the ends of the roll in a certain angle and affix it to the side of a log. Dust it with some cocoa powder and serve.

II.   Coconut Flour Cake

Ingredients:

For the cake:

- ¾ cups of honey

- 2 teaspoons of vanilla extract

- 2 cups of coconut milk

- ½ teaspoon of baking soda

- ¼ teaspoon of unrefined sea salt

- ½ teaspoon of coconut extract

- 2 cups of coconut flour

- ½ teaspoon of orange extract

- Coconut oil

For the frosting:

- 2 cups coconut spread

- ½ cup of virgin coconut oil

- 1/3 cup of honey

- 1 teaspoon of vanilla extract

- 1 teaspoon of coconut extract

Instructions:

1. Preheat the oven to 350 degrees F.

2. Take a large bowl. Beat the eggs along with the coconut milk, honey, vanilla, coconut extract and orange extract. Keep beating till the mixture turns smooth and creamy.

3. Add the coconut flour to the bowl and mix well.

4. Add the baking soda and unrefined sea salt to the bowl and mix well. Keep mixing till the consistency of the batter is smooth.

5. Now, take an 8-inch cake tin and grease them well.

6. Now fill the cake tin with the batter. Ensure that the batter is spread evenly.

7. Place the tin in the oven and bake the cake for around forty minutes. This should be sufficient time for the cake to get cooked and get separated from the sides of the tins. To check if the cake has cooked well, insert a toothpick into the cake. If it comes out clean, the cake is good to go.

8. Remove the cake from the oven and allow it to cool.

9. As the cake is cooling, let's get started with the coconut frosting. Take a small bowl. Add the coconut oil, vanilla extract, coconut spread, honey and coconut extract to the bowl and whisk well. Keep whisking till the ingredients combine well and soft peaks form.

10. Place the frosting in the refrigerator for around ten minutes. This should be sufficient time for the frosting to stiffen.

11. At the end of ten minutes, remove the frosting from the oven. Beat it well for a minute.

12. Once the cake has cooled enough, invert it over a kitchen towel slowly.

13. Proceed to spread the coconut frosting on the cake. Place the cake on a serving platter, with its seam down.

III.   Chocolate Mint Mousse

Ingredients:

- 4 whole eggs

- 1 tablespoon of vanilla extract

- ¼ teaspoon of mint extract

- 1 cup of cocoa powder

- 1 ¼ cup of cream or whole milk

- 1 handful of mint leaves

- ¼ teaspoon of unrefined sea salt

- ¼ cup of whole and unrefined cane sugar

Instructions:

1. Wash the mint leaves well. Keep aside a few for garnishing and crush the remaining leaves. This will release most of the flavors, which will otherwise be lost if you mince or chop it.

2. Take a large pot. Add the cream or whole milk into it. Heat it over a low flame. When the temperature increases, remove the pot from the heat.

3.   Add the crushed leaves to the pot and allow them to rest in the cream for at least half an hour.

4.   At the end of thirty minutes, remove the mint leaves and place the pot on the stove again. Keep heating it over a medium low heat.

5.   Now, add the eggs to the pot and mix well.

6.   Add the cocoa powder and salt to the pot next. Keep whisking till all the ingredients are mixed well.

7.   Keep cooking the mixture in the stove over medium low heat till the consistency of the mousse is thick. Keep whisking continuously to ensure that the mousse thickens.

8.   When the mousse reaches the consistency akin to a pudding, remove the pot from the heat. Add in the mint extract and vanilla extract and mix well.

9.   Allow the mixture to cool for some time.

10.   Once the mousse has cooled enough, transfer it to serving bowls. Garnish with the remaining mint leaves and serve.

IV.   Olive Oil Ice Cream

Ingredients:

- 1 ½ cups of unrefined, extra virgin olive oil

- 4 cups of whole milk

- 4 cups of heavy cream

- 4 blood oranges

- 12 egg yolks, beaten

- Pinch of unrefined sea salt

- 1 cup of raw honey

- 12 to 16 drops of orange essential oil

Instructions:

1.   Take the oranges first. Grate their skins and keep the zest aside.

2.   Now, take out the orange segments. Remove the membranes and piths. Place the orange segments in a small bowl.

3.   Take a medium sized bowl. Add the olive oil, whole milk, heavy cream and beaten eggs to it. Whisk well till the ingredients combine well and begin to emulsify.

4.   Now, add in the raw honey and whisk vigorously. If your eggs and milk are cold, the honey might harden. This will make it difficult for you to mix the honey with the milk mixture. To ensure that the honey blends in well, pour the egg and milk mixture into a saucepan and heat it over a low heat. Whisk in the honey as the egg mixture begins warming up.

5.   Now, add in the orange zest, unrefined sea salt and orange essential oil and mix well.

6.   If you have warmed the egg mixture, allow it to cool. Place the mixture in the refrigerator for around 20 minutes. This should be sufficient time for the mixture to cool down.

7.   At the end of twenty minutes, remove the mixture from the refrigerator. Fold in the orange segments.

8.   Return the bowl back to the refrigerator and let it cool for around one to two hours. Let your ice cream base chill for some time.

9.   At the end of two hours, remove the bowl from the refrigerator and transfer the base to the ice cream churner. Follow the instructions given on your ice cream maker to prepare it. Serve cold.

V.   Maple Pecan Pie

Ingredients:

- 1 ½ cups of pecan halves

- 1 ½ cups of sifted and sprouted spelt flour

- ½ teaspoon of unrefined sea salt

- ½ cup of cold water

- 4 eggs

- ¾ cup of cold lard, chopped into smaller pieces

- ½ cup of whole and unrefined cane sugar

- 2 tablespoons of butter, melted

- 1 cup of maple syrup

- 1 tablespoon of vanilla bean powder

Instructions:

1.   Preheat the oven to 350 degrees F.

2.   Take a stand mixer. Add the flour and salt to it and whisk them well. Add the chopped lard next and whisk. Keep whisking till the consistency of the mixture is that of corn meal. Now,

remove the whisk attachment and attach the dough hook. Add in the cold water slowly as the flour is getting processed. Keep processing till dough is formed and it stops sticking to the sides of the bowl.

3.   Now, remove the dough from the mixer. Place it between two pieces of parchment papers and roll it out. Keep rolling till its thickness is 1/8 inch.

4.   Take a 9 inch pie pan. Place the disc of the dough in it. Place the pan in the refrigerator and let it rest.

5.   As the dough is resting, let's get started with the remaining ingredients. Take a large bowl. First, beat the eggs well with the cane sugar.

6.   Now add the maple syrup, vanilla bean powder and melted butter to the bowl and mix well.

7.   Now, remove the pie crust from the freezer. Pour in the filling.

8.   Arrange the pecan halves on top of the filling. Ensure that the pecan halves are soaked well overnight and dehydrated.

9.   Place the crust in the oven and bake it for around forty minutes. This should be sufficient time for the crust to turn golden and the center to remain wobbly.

10.   Remove the pie from the oven and allow it to cool before serving.

VI.   Sugar Plums

Ingredients:

- 2 cups of shelled walnuts

- 1 teaspoon unrefined sea salt

- zest of 2 oranges

- 2 teaspoons of ground cinnamon

- 1 teaspoon of finely grated nutmeg

- ½ teaspoon of ground allspice

- ½ teaspoon of ground coriander

- 2 cups of finely chopped dates, pits removed

- 1 apricot, finely chopped

- 1 cup of finely chopped prunes, pits removed

- Powdered unrefined cane sugar, optional

- Unsweetened desiccated coconut

- Warm water

Instructions:

1.   Take a large mixing bowl. Add the walnuts to the bowl followed by the unrefined sea salt.

2.   Pour some warm water into the bowl. Cover the bowl with a lid and allow the nuts to soak in the salt infused water for any time between eight and twelve hours. You can let the nuts soak overnight to save some preparation time.

3.   Once the nuts have soaked enough, transfer them to a colander to drain the water. Rinse them well with some water. Use a kitchen towel to pat the nuts dry.

4.   Now, add the soaked nuts to the bowl of a food processor.

5.   Add the orange zest, allspice, grated nutmeg, ground cinnamon, chopped dates, ground coriander, chopped prunes and chopped apricot to the food processor.

6.   Pulse the mixture at least three to four times. This should be sufficient for the ingredients to combine well. Keep processing till a fine paste is formed from the dry fruits, spices and walnuts.

7.   Take another large mixing bowl. Transfer the paste to the bowl. Let's get started with the sugar plums. Take two tablespoons of the paste and start rolling it in the center of your

palms. Keep rolling till you make a round ball out of the paste in hand. Ensure that the entire paste is rolled out into similar balls.

8.   Dust the sugar plums with powdered unrefined cane sugar and allow it to rest for a few minutes. This should be sufficient time for the sugar to settle.

9.   Garnish the sugar plums with the desiccated coconut and serve.

VII.   Mangoes With Sticky Rice

Ingredients:

- 2 tablespoons of lime juice

- 28 ounces of full fat coconut milk

- 2 cups of short grain brown rice

- 2 teaspoons of unrefined sea salt

- ½ cup of coconut oil

- 2 ripe mangoes

- 4 tablespoons of coconut palm sugar or unrefined cane sugar

- zest of 2 limes

- Water

Instructions:

1.   Wash the mangoes well. Peel their skins off. Using a sharp knife, slice the mangoes thinly.

2.   Take the brown rice in a large bowl. Place it under a running tap and rinse it well. Once the grains are rinsed well, drain the water.

3.   Pour some warm water into the bowl and let the rice soak in it.

4.   Now, add the lime juice to the bowl and stir well. Let the rice soak in this acidic water for at least 8 to 12 hours.

5.   At the end of twelve hours, drain the rice. Rinse it again using water before you start cooking the rice.

6.   Measure the rice and place it in the cooking pot. Add 4 ½ cups of water to the cooking pot.

7.   Read the instructions manual and cook the rice in the cooker. Do not keep lifting the lid to check if the rice is cooked. This will increase the cooking time.

8.   As the rice is cooking in the cooker, take a medium sized saucepan. Add the full fat coconut milk to the saucepan and heat it over a medium low heat.

9.   Now, add the unrefined sea salt and unrefined cane sugar to the saucepan and mix. Keep mixing till the salt and the sugar dissolve completely in the milk. Remove the saucepan from the heat.

10.   Once the rice is cooked, remove the cooker from the heat and transfer the cooked rice to a large bowl. Let the steam settle for a few minutes.

11.   Pour half the coconut milk mixture over the cooked rice and mix.

12.   Now, pour the coconut oil on top of the contents of the bowl. Allow the rice mixture to rest for around twenty minutes. This should be sufficient time for the rice to soak in the coconut oil.

13.   Divide the rice between 12 serving bowls. Pour the remaining coconut milk mixture over the rice.

14.   Now, arrange the mango slices neatly on top of the rice.

15.   Garnish the bowls with lime zest. Serve warm.

VIII. Cinnamon Molasses Cookies

Ingredients:

- 2 cups of grass-fed butter, softened

- 2 cups of whole, unrefined cane sugar

- 1 cup of blackstrap molasses

- 4 pastured eggs, beaten

- 2 teaspoons of vanilla extract

- 8 cups of sprouted grain flour

- 1 teaspoon of unrefined sea salt

- 4 teaspoons of baking soda

- 4 tablespoons of ground cinnamon

Instructions:

1. Take a small bowl. Add the cream and sugar to the bowl and mix well. Keep mixing till they combine well and turn light and fluffy.

2. Now, add the molasses and vanilla extract to the cream mixture slowly. Keep beating till the ingredients combine well.

3.   Now, add the beaten eggs to the bowl. Keep mixing to ensure that the eggs combine well with the cream mixture.

4.   Take another bowl. Add the unrefined sea salt, sprouted flour, ground cinnamon and baking soda to the bowl. Mix well.

5.   Now, mix the flour mixture with the cream mixture. Keep mixing till the wet ingredients combine well with the dry ingredients.

6.   Place the dough in the refrigerator and allow it to rest for at least four hours.

7.   As the dough is resting, preheat the oven to 350 degrees F.

8.   As the oven is getting heated, take a small bowl. Add around 4 tablespoons of unrefined cane sugar, ground cinnamon and unrefined sea salt to the bowl. Mix well.

9.   Let's get started with the dough balls. Take two tablespoons of the cookie dough and start rolling it in the center of your palms. Keep rolling till you make a ball out of the paste in hand. Ensure that the entire dough is rolled out into similar balls.

10.   Roll the dough balls in the cinnamon topping.

11. Now, arrange the dough balls on the preheated baking stone. To ensure that the balls are evenly spread, press down with the tines of a fork.

12. Bake the cookies in the oven for at least six to eight times. This should be sufficient time for the cookies to get baked thoroughly and turn crisp. Remove the cookies from the oven at the end of eight minutes. Serve warm.

Closing Thoughts & What You Need To Do Next!

Thank you again for purchasing this book!

I hope this book was able to help you to understand and embrace the alternatives of healing through natural remedies and eating the proper food as a way to combat Inflammation.

The next step is to gradually eliminate the foods that are bad for you and incorporate alternative solutions that suit the Anti-Inflammatory Diet.

Finally, if you enjoyed this book, then I'd like to ask you for a favour, would you be kind enough to leave a review for this book on Amazon? It'd be greatly appreciated!

Type the link below into your browser to leave a review.

www.amazon.com/product-reviews/B00YT0JK12

Thank You & Good Luck!

Other Books By This Author

Lactose Intolerance: Going Dairy Free - Reduce The Effects of Milk, Allergies & Food Intolerances

http://www.amazon.com/gp/product/B019ALCAR0

How do you eliminate Lactose from your diet? What can you do to get the nutrition you need?

This book will help you clean out your digestive system, experiment with non-dairy foods and drinks, and change your lifestyle for the better. You'll discover how to get the **calcium and other nutrients** your body requires - and how to replace the foods you can't tolerate with a huge variety of healthy options!

Get Instant Access To Your FREE BONUS Gift by signing up for our Health Newsletter

FREE BONUS Ebook

"Top 10 Tips to Naturally Supercharge Your Health & Vitality"

https://publishfunnel.leadpages.co/free-top-10-health-vitality-tips/

Join Our Book Club To Get Our Best Kindle Books For FREE!

FREE BONUS Ebook

"Stress Buster Formula - Hidden Blueprint Code"

https://publishfunnel.leadpages.co/resolute-minds-publishing-book-club/

Made in the USA
Lexington, KY
02 November 2017